Workbook

to Accompany

Principles of Radiographic Imaging

An Art and a Science

6th Edition

Workbook
to Accompany
Principles of Radiographic Imaging
An Art and a Science

6th Edition

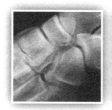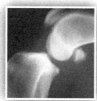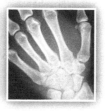

Revised by
Debra J. Poelhuis, MS, RT(R)(M)
Director, Radiography Program
Montgomery County Community College
Pottstown, Pennsylvania

Nina Kowalczyk, PhD, RT(R)(CT)(QM), FASRT
Assistant Professor—Radiologic Sciences and Therapy
School of Allied Medical Professions
The Ohio State University
Columbus, Ohio

❄ Cengage

Australia • Brazil • Canada • Mexico • Singapore • United Kingdom • United States

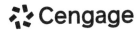

Workbook to Accompany Principles of Radiographic Imaging: An Art and a Science, Sixth Edition
Debra J. Poelhuis and
Nina Kowalczyk

SVP, GM Skills & Global Product Management: Jonathan Lau

Product Director: Matthew Seeley

Product Team Manager: Stephen Smith

Product Manager: Lauren Whalen

Product Assistant: Jessica Molesky

Executive Director, Content Design: Marah Bellegarde

Director, Learning Design: Juliet Steiner

Learning Designer: Deborah Bordeaux

Vice President, Marketing Services: Jennifer Ann Baker

Marketing Director: Sean Chamberland

Marketing Manager: Jonathan Sheehan

Senior Director, Content Delivery: Wendy Troeger

Senior Content Manager: Thomas Heffernan

Digital Delivery Lead: Derek Allison

Managing Art Director: Jack Pendleton

Senior Designer: Angela Sheehan

Cover Images: Xray Computer/Shutterstock.com

Production Service/Compositor: SPi Global

For product information and technology assistance, contact us at
**Cengage Customer & Sales Support, 1-800-354-9706
or support.cengage.com.**

For permission to use material from this text or product, submit all requests online at **www.copyright.com**.

Example: Microsoft® is a registered trademark of the Microsoft Corporation.

Library of Congress Control Number: 2018964618

ISBN: 978-1-337-79311-7

Cengage
200 Pier 4 Boulevard
Boston, MA 02210
USA

Cengage is a leading provider of customized learning solutions with employees residing in nearly 40 different countries and sales in more than 125 countries around the world. Find your local representative at: **www.cengage.com**.

To learn more about Cengage platforms and services, register or access your online learning solution, or purchase materials for your course, visit **www.cengage.com**.

Notice to the Reader
Publisher does not warrant or guarantee any of the products described herein or perform any independent analysis in connection with any of the product information contained herein. Publisher does not assume, and expressly disclaims, any obligation to obtain and include information other than that provided to it by the manufacturer. The reader is expressly warned to consider and adopt all safety precautions that might be indicated by the activities described herein and to avoid all potential hazards. By following the instructions contained herein, the reader willingly assumes all risks in connection with such instructions. The publisher makes no representations or warranties of any kind, including but not limited to, the warranties of fitness for particular purpose or merchantability, nor are any such representations implied with respect to the material set forth herein, and the publisher takes no responsibility with respect to such material. The publisher shall not be liable for any special, consequential, or exemplary damages resulting, in whole or part, from the readers' use of, or reliance upon, this material.

Printed in the United States of America
Print Number: 06   Print Year: 2022

Dedicated to

Noah and Elizabeth Holdorf
William Leth
Nick Kowalczyk

In Memory of

Frank and Irene Marcoccia

Contents

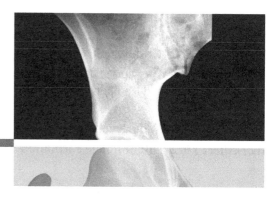

UNIT IV Digital Radiography Introduction

UNIT V Analyzing the Image

UNIT VI Special Imaging Systems and Modalities

Preface

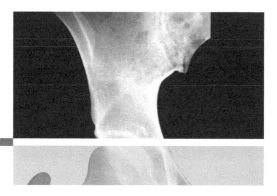

This workbook has been designed to correlate with the textbook *Principles of Radiographic Imaging: An Art and a Science,* 6th edition. Our intent has been to design a series of exercises, both laboratories and worksheets, to provide higher-level synthesis and analysis activities for each chapter in the textbook. There are 80 exercises, of which 48 are laboratories and 32 are worksheets. There is at least one exercise for most text chapter, with multiple activities for chapters that require exercises to assist students in understanding the more difficult concepts. Linear and semilog graph paper masters are included at the end of the workbook for use where applicable.

This workbook represents a correlated series of exercises to help strengthen didactic instruction. There are sufficient activities to support a regularly scheduled laboratory for courses in physics, principles of exposure, and imaging. An equipment chart is provided to assist faculty in preparing for each laboratory and for ordering supplies and equipment prior to each course.

Students are expected to be able to operate radiographic equipment as well as a processor, densitometer, sensitometer, oscilloscope, and ion chamber dosimeter for various exercises. No worksheets or laboratories are provided to teach students the operation of this equipment, since we found wide differences in manufacturers'

operating instructions. We suggest that students be shown how to operate each new piece of equipment at the start of the laboratory where it must be used. Alternatively, faculty may produce laboratory exercises for this purpose by duplicating the relevant portions of the manufacturer's operating manual.

Many of the exercises in this workbook were based on laboratories that have been in use for many years at The Ohio State University, Rhodes State College, and Indiana University Northwest. Other exercises were designed specifically for the chapters in the textbook. All of the activities were tested and found to be sound in concept. Additional testing was done by Barry Burns at the University of North Carolina. Each activity has a set of instructions with reasonable equipment requirements and preparation time.

We acknowledge responsibility for all errors in content. It is the responsibility of faculty to properly prepare students for laboratory coursework, and therefore we assume no responsibility for damage to equipment or persons as a result of students performing these exercises. In addition, information in this workbook should only be used in clinical practice subservient to prevailing procedures and under the direction of appropriate supervisory personnel.

Exposure Technique Factors

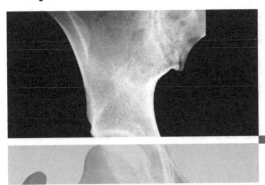

The use of these laboratories requires fine adjustment of exposure technical factors for each exercise. Most of the experiments that use radiographic film are based on the use of a CR imaging system. Since film is no longer the imaging system of choice, some experiments have included instructions for film/screen, CR or DR imaging. Because of the complex variations in diagnostic imaging systems, it is impossible to suggest exposure factors that will produce ideal results in all situations. Faculty members may wish to produce the images for each experiment in order to obtain exact technical factors prior to assigning the laboratories to students. Alternately, if students are working individually or in small groups, the entire group may learn valuable lessons by assisting in adjusting our suggested factors until an ideal exposure has been achieved for each activity. In all cases, the **exposure should be adjusted by mAs changes only** (unless otherwise stated in the laboratory instructions). **Kilovoltage levels have been chosen for specific effects in many experiments and should not be changed unless absolutely necessary due to equipment limitations.**

Laboratory Equipment and Materials

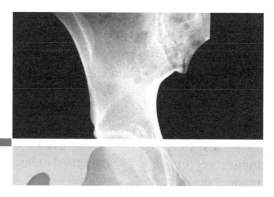

The majority of laboratory activities contained in this manual require specific items that are common to a radiography environment. In order to facilitate the instructor and student in preparing for the laboratory activities, the following equipment/materials matrix lists the basic equipment and materials requirements for each laboratory experiment. For a more complete description of the recommended items, the reader should refer to the specific laboratory experiment. Laboratory materials listed with a # sign indicate items with alternative choices or options for completion of the experiment. Those listed with a * sign indicate that the items have to be prepared or constructed prior to the experiment. Refer to the specific experiment for detailed instructions. Keep in mind that the equipment/materials recommendations have been made based on field trials and are not etched in stone, so feel free to substitute the equipment and/or material items if deemed necessary. Remember that ingenuity is the mother of all experiments.

3-1	**3-2**	**4-1**	**4-2**
Electroscope	1.5-V battery (5) or DC power source	#9-V battery (dry cell)	Bar magnets (different strengths)
Static rods	Ammeter/Voltmeter	Bar magnets	Galvanometer or ammeter
Silk patches	Copper wire	Cardboard, stiff paper, Plexiglass (8 × 10)	*Wire helix coils
Wool patches	Resistors (five 5-watt)	Compass	Copper wire with alligator clips
		Galvanometer or ammeter	
		Iron filings	
		Wire (3′)	

5-1	**9-1**	**10-1**	**11-1**
X-ray tube parts	Ionization Chamber Dosimeter	Ionization Chamber Dosimeter	Radiographic unit
	Phantom body part	Gonad shields	Four 1-mm Al attenuators
	Radiographic unit	Phantom body part	Ionization Chamber Dosimeter
	Ring stand	Radiographic unit	Semi-log graph paper
		Ring stand	

11-2
0.25-, 0.5-, 1.0-,
   2.0-mm Al filters
Radiographic unit
Ionization Chamber
   Dosimeter

12-2
Ionization Chamber
   Dosimeter
Radiographic unit

13-1
Cassette/image
   receptor
Ionization Chamber
   Dosimeter
Image processor
Phantom body part
Radiographic unit

14-1
Digital dosimeter
Radiographic unit
Technique chart

15-1
Image receptor
Image processor
Phantom body part
Plastic gallon jugs
Radiographic unit

16-1
Energized radiographic
   unit
Chest phantom
Ionization Chamber
   Dosimeter
Image processor

17-1
Image receptor—
   digital and/or film
   screen
Cassette holder
Ionization Chamber
   Dosimeter
Image processor
Phantom body part
Radiographic unit
Wire mesh tool
Densitometer

17-2
Teaching radiographic
   images

18-1
Aluminum step wedge
Image receptor
Densitometer
Image processor
Phantom body part
8:1 and 12:1 grids
Radiographic unit

18-2
Image receptor
Image processor
Phantom body part
12:1 grid
Radiographic unit

18-3
Radiographic unit
Image receptor
Phantom
8:1 and 12:1 grids (2)

20-2
Radiographic unit
CR or DR image
   receptor
Image processor
Phantom

20-3
CR or DR imaging
   system
Image processor
Phantom body part

21-1
Radiographic unit
CR cassettes
Phantom body part
Image processor

25-1
Radiographic unit
Phantom body part
Cassette
CR cassettes or DR unit
   film processor
CR image processor
Film processor

26-1
Aluminum step wedge
Cassette/image
   receptor
Image processor
Phantom body part
Radiographic unit

26-2

Aluminum step wedge
Cassette/image
  receptor
Image processor
Phantom body part
Radiographic unit

26-3

Cassette/image
  receptor
Densitometer
Film processor
Phantom body part
Radiographic unit
CR image processor
CR cassettes

26-4

Aluminum step wedge
Image receptor
Densitometer
Image processor
Phantom body part
Radiographic unit

26-6

1″ super ball
35-mm film canister
Barium solution
3″ to 4″ container
Image receptor
Image processor
Ice cubes
Radiographic unit
Note: These images
  are also used for
  Laboratory 27-2

27-1

Aluminum step wedge
Image receptors
Densitometer
Image processor
Phantom body part
Radiographic unit

27-2

Use films/supplies from
  Laboratory 26-6

27-3

Cassette/image
  receptor
Image processor
Phantom body part
Radiographic unit

27-4

Aluminum step wedge
Cassette/image
  receptor
Densitometer
Image processor
Phantom body part
Radiographic grids
Radiographic unit

28-1

Image receptor
Dry bones
Image processor
Radiographic unit
Resolution test pattern
Sponges
Lead masks

28-2

Image receptor
Dry bones
Image processor
Radiographic unit
Resolution test pattern
Sponges

28-3

CR image receptor
Image processor
Phantom body part
Radiographic unit
String

29-1

Image receptor
Small dry bone
  (vertebrae preferred)
Image processor
Metric ruler
Radiographic unit

29-2

Image receptors
Dry bones
Image processor
Metric ruler
Radiographic unit

30-1

Repeated images

31-1

Image receptor
Image processor
Metric ruler
Radiographic unit
Star test pattern

31-2

Beam perpendicularity
  test tool
Image receptors
#Collimator test tool
Image processor
Nine pennies
Radiographic unit with
  PBL
Cardboard
Paper clips

31-3

Image receptor
Image processor
Metric ruler
Radiographic unit
Ring stand
Paper sheet protector
  for 8 × 11 paper
Bubble level
Angulator
Quarter or other coin

31-4

Digital kVp meter
Image processor
kVp test cassette (with
  current calibration
  chart)
Radiographic unit

31-5

Image receptor
Image processor
Protractor
Radiographic unit
Digital exposure timer

31-6

Digital dosimeter
Radiographic unit

31-7

Rejected images
Rejected analysis
  worksheet

33-1

Fluoroscopic unit
Lead apron
Phantom body part

32-1

Image receptor
Image processor
Coconut
Mobile Radiographic
  unit

33-1

Fluoroscopic unit
Lead apron
Phantom body part

39-2

CT images, abdomen
MR images, abdomen

40-2

Nuclear medicine
  images

42-2

Ultrasound images

UNIT I Creating the Beam

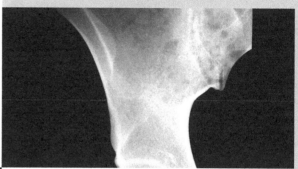

WORKSHEET 1–1 BASIC MATHEMATICS REVIEW

PURPOSE

Drill and practice in solving basic mathematical problems.

FOR FURTHER REVIEW

Refer to Chapter 1 in the accompanying textbook for further review of this topic.

ACTIVITIES

Carry out the math operations indicated and solve the following problems:

Problems for Fractions

1. $1/9 + 4/9 =$

2. $4/9 - 2/9 =$

3. $2/5 \div 3/4 =$

4. $3/4 \cdot 1/5 =$

5. $2/3 \div 5/7 =$

Problems for Decimals

1. $(34.21) \cdot (1.1) =$

2. $714.58 + 214.785 =$

3. $725 \div 0.25 =$

4. Change 85 percent to a decimal.

5. Change 0.081 to a percent.

Problems for Computation with Values (Numbers)

1. Round each of the following to the number of significant digits indicated.

    a. 328.14 (4)

    b. 1.25   (2)

    c. 2,709 (3)

2. Multiply or divide the following numbers, leaving the result with the correct number of significant digits if each number is assumed to be approximate.

   a. (2.32)(1.2)

   b. (43.81) ÷ (2.23)

3. Multiply or divide the following numbers, leaving the result with the correct number of significant digits if each number is assumed to be approximate.

   a. (38.42)(3.82)

   b. (4.32) ÷ (1.5)

4. Add or subtract the following numbers, leaving the result with the correct number of significant digits if each number is assumed to be approximate.

   a. 21.3 + 21.39

   b. 48.61 + 61

5. How many significant digits are in each of the following?

   a. 7.04

   b. 180

   c. 180.0

   d. 9,300

   e. 8,104.6

Problems with Powers of 10

1. Solve the following:

   a. 82×10^4

   b. 18×10^3

   c. 14×10^2

Problems for Scientific Notation

1. Change the following numbers to scientific notation.

   a. 784.2

   b. 0.00431

   c. 78,210,000

   d. 0.0000067

   e. 7.4

WORKSHEET 1-1 (Continued)

2. Change the following numbers to ordinary notation.

    a. 2.84×10^5

    b. 2.84×10^{-5}

    c. 6.18×10^0

    d. 6.18×10^{-2}

    e. 6.18×10^1

Problems for Signed Numbers

1. $(-6) - (-9) + (-6) =$

2. $(-8)(-2)(-3) =$

3. $(15) \div (-13) =$

4. $-6 - 8 - 2 + 3 =$

5. $(-2)(-1)(-1)(-1) =$

Problems for Order of Operation

1. Evaluate each of the following:

    a. $17 - 8.2 + 4 \cdot 5 - 2.6^2$

    b. $(3 + 1)^2 - 4(8 + 2) - 5 \cdot (-1)$

    c. $6(2^2 - 4 \cdot 1) - 4^2$

    d. $-2(3 + 4 \cdot 5)$

    e. $(-8)^2 + 3 \cdot 5^2$

2. Evaluate each of the following:

    a. $7 + 4 \cdot 5$

    b. $6 \cdot 7 - 4 \cdot (-6)$

    c. $2 \cdot 7^2$

    d. $(-4)^2$

    e. -4^2

    f. $6(7 + 3) + 4 \cdot 8 - 7^2$

Problems for Algebraic Expressions

1. Simplify the following algebraic expressions.

    a. $2(3x + 4y) + (x - y)$

    b. $2(x - 4y) - 6(x + 2y)$

    c. $6[2x - 4(x - y)]$

    d. $-3[2(x + 5y) - 6(2x + 3y)]$

2. Simplify the following algebraic expressions.

    a. $2(3x + 4y) + (x - y)$

    b. $3(x - 2y) - 6(x + y)$

    c. $4[3x - 2(2x - 3y)]$

    d. $8[-2(2x + 3) + 4(x - y)]$

Problems for Exponents

1. Simplify each of the following expressions, leaving the answer with only positive exponents.

    a. $a^4 \cdot a^5 \cdot a^3$

    b. $\dfrac{b^8 \cdot b^4}{b^5}$

    c. $(a^2)^3 (b^{-2})^{-5}$

    d. $\dfrac{a^4 b^2 a^8 b^6}{a^5 b^3 a^{10} b^2}$

WORKSHEET 1–1 (Continued)

2. Simplify each of the following expressions, leaving the answer with only positive exponents.

a. $a^2 \cdot a^4 \cdot a^8$

b. $\dfrac{b^6 \, b^2}{b^5}$

c. $a^2 \cdot b^5 \cdot a^5 \cdot b^2$

d. $\dfrac{a^8 b^{10}}{a^{11} b^4}$

Problems for Evaluating Algebraic Expressions

1. Evaluate each of the following expressions for $a = 5$, $b = 3$, and $c = -2$.

a. $a + b \cdot c$

b. $a + b - c$

c. $2c + 3b^2 + 2(a - c)$

2. Evaluate each of the following expressions for $a = 2$, $b = -4$, and $c = 6$.

a. $2a + 3b - 4c$

b. $b^2 - 2c^2 + a^2$

c. $5(a + 2b - c) + 4 \cdot b$

Problems for Equations

1. Solve for x: $x/6 = 3$

2. Solve for y: $2y + 3 = 9$

3. Solve for b: $2(b + 6) = b + 12$

4. Solve for x: $18/11 = 3/x$

5. Solve for a: $3(a + 4) = 15$

Problems for Variation

1. If y varies directly as x, and x = 9 when y = 15, find y when x = 33.

2. If c varies directly as the square root of d, and c = 14 when d = 64, find c when d = 324.

3. If y varies inversely as x, and y = 32 when x = 3, find x when y = 15.

WORKSHEET 1-2 UNITS OF MEASUREMENT

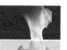

PURPOSE

Drill and practice in solving units of measurement and dimensional analysis problems.

FOR FURTHER REVIEW

Refer to Chapter 1 in the accompanying textbook for further review of this topic.

ACTIVITIES

Carry out the math operations indicated and solve the following problems:

Problems for Dimensional Analysis

Convert the following:

1. 15 inches to yards

2. 1,500 seconds to hours

3. 1.8 hours to seconds

4. 18.9 feet to inches

5. 60 miles/hour to feet/second

6. 44 feet/second to miles/hour

7. 10 feet^2 to inches^2

8. 10 meters^2 to centimeters^2

9. 14 inches^3 to feet^3

10. 15 yards^3 to feet^3

11. 15.8 g/cm^3 to kg/m^3

12. 6.8 gallons to pints

WORKSHEET 1-2 (Continued)

Identify the SI unit of measurement and symbol for the following quantities:

Quantity	Unit	Symbol
13. Length	_____	_____
14. Mass	_____	_____
15. Time	_____	_____
16. Exposure	_____	_____
17. Absorbed Dose	_____	_____
18. Dose Equivalent	_____	_____

Convert the following:

19. 500 milliroentgens to coulombs/kilogram

20. 20 millirem to sieverts

21. 50 rads to grays

22. 6.45×10^{-4} coulombs/kilogram to roentgens

23. 0.084 sievert to rems

24. 0.35 gray to rads

LABORATORY 3-1 LAWS OF ELECTROSTATICS AND ELECTRODYNAMICS

PURPOSE

Interpret the results of various electrostatic interactions.

FOR FURTHER REVIEW

Refer to Chapter 3 in the accompanying textbook for further review of this topic.

MATERIALS

1. Electroscope

2. Static conducting rods or plastic strips

3. Small pieces of wool and silk

PROCEDURES

1. Always ground the electroscope by gently touching the knob with the palm of your hand prior to performing any experiment. If your electroscope has thin metal leaves, never touch them.

2. Use a piece of cloth to rub your conducting strip, then touch the knob of the electroscope. Record your observations. Repeat for each type of cloth available.

3. Use a piece of cloth to rub your conducting strip, then bring the conducting strip close to, but do not allow it to touch, the knob of the electroscope. Record your observations. Repeat for each type of cloth available.

RESULTS

1. Record the reaction that was observed in the electroscope for each type of cloth when the conducting rod or strip touched the knob.

2. Record the reaction that was observed in the electroscope for each type of cloth when the conducting rod or strip came near, but did not touch, the knob.

ANALYSIS

Use two + signs to indicate the presence of electrons. Do not use any − signs.

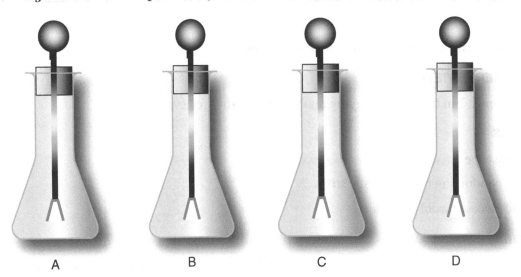

1. Use Figure A to indicate the distribution of electrons and the position of the leaves while a charged conducting rod was in contact with the knob.

2. Use Figure B to indicate the distribution of electrons and the position of the leaves after a charged rod was removed from contact with the knob.

3. Use Figure C to indicate the distribution of electrons and the position of the leaves while a charged rod was near, but not touching, the knob.

4. Use Figure D to indicate the distribution of electrons and the position of the leaves after a charged rod was removed from proximity with the knob.

5. Were there any differences in the effect seen with the various cloths? Why?

6. Which law of electrostatics was demonstrated in Figure A?

7. What is the term for the effect seen in Figure B?

8. What effect would be seen if the electroscope was subjected to an intense dose of ionizing radiation?

Name _____ Course _____ Date _____

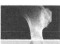 **LABORATORY 3-2** OHM'S LAW AND RESISTANCE

PURPOSE

Demonstrate the relationships involved in Ohm's law.

FOR FURTHER REVIEW

Refer to Chapter 3 in the accompanying textbook for further review of this topic.

MATERIALS

1. DC variable power source (five 1.5-V C or D size batteries can be substituted)

2. Five 10-Ω, 5-watt resistors

3. Meters capable of measuring 0 to 10 V and 0 to 1,000 mA (0–1 A)

4. Connecting wires

PROCEDURES

Effect of EMF on Current Flow

1. Connect two 10-Ω resistors in series and hook the combination in series with an ammeter and the power source. Use a voltmeter across the power source to set it at 1.5 V. Record the applied voltage and the current flow as measured by the ammeter (in the range of 75 mA).

2. Repeat step 1 four more times after increasing the voltage in increments of 1.5 V up to a total of 7.5 V while leaving the resistance the same.

Effect of Resistance on Current Flow

1. Use a voltmeter connected across the power source to adjust it to 6 V. Connect one 10-Ω resistor in series with the ammeter and hook the combination in series with the power source. Record the current measured by the ammeter (in the range of 600 mA).

2. Repeat step 1 for resistance values of 20, 30, 40, and 50 Ω by connecting in turn two, three, four, and five of the 10-Ω resistors in series.

LABORATORY 3-2 (Continued)

Effect of Voltage on Current Flow

1. Plot the following graph of current (I) against applied voltage (V) using the data obtained from steps 1 and 2. (Mark the vertical axis with mA values that will permit all your data to be graphed.)

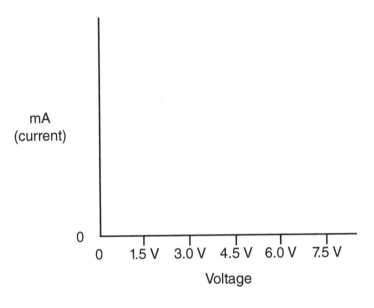

Effect of Resistance on Current Flow

1. Plot the following graph of current (I) against resistance (R) using the data obtained from steps 1 and 2. (Mark the vertical axis with mA values that will permit all your data to be graphed.)

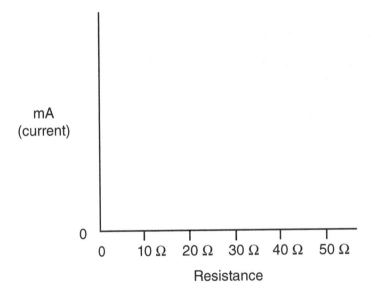

LABORATORY 3-2 (Continued)

ANALYSIS

Ohm's Law

Use Ohm's law to fill in the missing quantities in the chart.

	Amps	Volts	Ohms
1.	100	_____	4
2.	56	_____	312
3.	_____	110	60
4.	_____	2,110	11.5
5.	50	110	_____
6.	0.8	39	_____

Effect of Series and Parallel Circuits on Resistance, Current, and emf

7. What is the total resistance of a circuit if it contains resistances of 3 Ω, 2 Ω, and 10 Ω in series? in parallel?

8. What is the total resistance of a circuit if it contains resistances of 110 Ω, 26.2 Ω, and 14 Ω in series? in parallel?

9. If a circuit has resistances of 10 Ω, 12 Ω, and 2.4 Ω and an emf of 140 V, what is the current if the circuit has the resistances in series? in parallel?

10. If a circuit has resistances of 10 Ω, 4.2 Ω, and 3 Ω and a current of 56 amps, what is the emf if the circuit has the resistances in series? in parallel?

LABORATORY 3-2 (Continued)

Effect of Voltage on Current Flow

11. Based on the results of the experiment as shown on graph 1, when the resistance was relatively constant, what effect did voltage have on amperage? Is this finding consistent with Ohm's law?

Effect of Resistance on Current Flow

12. Based on the results of the experiment as shown on graph 2, when the voltage was relatively constant, what effect did resistance have on amperage? Is this finding consistent with Ohm's law?

LABORATORY 4-1 LAWS OF MAGNETISM AND MAGNETIC INDUCTION

PURPOSE

Demonstrate basic laws of magnetism, map static, and dynamic field flux lines, and illustrate the basic principle of magnetic induction.

FOR FURTHER REVIEW

Refer to Chapters 3 and 4 in the accompanying textbook for further review of this topic.

MATERIALS

1. Two bar magnets

2. Three pieces of stiff paper, cardboard, or Plexiglas (approximately 8" × 10")

3. Iron filings

4. 39 length of wire

5. Low-voltage power supply or dry cell (about 9 V)

6. Compass

7. Galvanometer (or ammeter)

PROCEDURES

Laws of Magnetism

1. Place the two bar magnets end to end with both S poles about 3" apart. Hold both magnets tightly and bring the two ends together.

2. Repeat step 1 with an N pole and an S pole together.

3. Repeat step 2 but hold the magnets away from each other at a distance of 2", 1", and 1/2" while feeling the force of the magnetic field at each distance. Record the distances in order of magnetic field strength.

Mapping a Static Field

1. Level the paper with spacers to permit the bar magnet to be positioned underneath.

2. Sprinkle the iron filings on the paper over the magnet.

Mapping a Dynamic Field

3. Run a wire vertically through a hole in the center of the paper (as shown in the figure). Connect the ends of a low-voltage battery (9-V dry cell suggested).

4. Draw arrows on the paper to map the direction of a compass needle (as shown in the textbook Figure 4-6). Place the compass on the surface of the paper and draw an arrow representing the direction of the compass needle. Slowly move the compass in a circle around the wire, adding arrows as the compass needle changes direction.

5. Reverse the connections of the wire at the battery and repeat step 4.

Magnetic Induction

6. Connect a wire (or wire coil) to an ammeter. Wave a bar magnet close to, but not touching, the wire while observing the meter.

ANALYSIS

Laws of Magnetism

1. Which law of magnetism was illustrated by steps 1 and 2?

2. Which law of magnetism was illustrated by step 3?

3. State the law of magnetism that would require breaking the bar magnets.

Mapping a Static Field

4. Draw the configuration of the magnetic lines of flux as revealed by the iron filings.

5. Why do the iron filings represent the magnetic lines of force?

Mapping a Dynamic Field

6. What is represented by the changing of the direction of the compass needle?

7. Explain the reason for the change in the direction of the lines of force between steps 4 and 5.

8. Which of the Fleming hand rules is demonstrated by this experiment?

9. Draw in the appropriate compass needle directions, lines of force directions, and electron flow on Figure A for one direction of flow and on Figure B for the other direction.

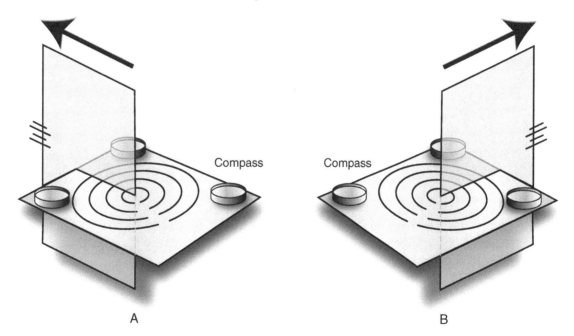

Compass   Compass

A   B

LABORATORY 4-1 (Continued)

Magnetic Induction

10. What effect does a moving magnetic field have on the current in a wire (or coil of wire)?

11. Explain (at the atomic level) how a moving magnetic field causes electrons to move along a wire, thus producing current through magnetic induction.

12. Add arrows in the appropriate direction for the induced magnetic field in the following Figure C.

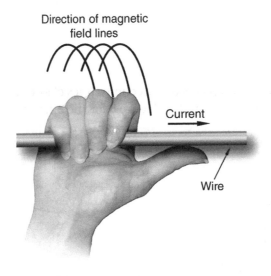

C

Name _____ Course _____ Date _____

 LABORATORY 4-2 ELECTROMAGNETIC INDUCTION

PURPOSE

Illustrate Faraday's laws of electromagnetics.

FOR FURTHER REVIEW

Refer to Chapter 4 in the accompanying textbook for further review of this topic.

MATERIALS

1. Helix coil of wire with few turns

2. Helix coil of wire with many turns

3. Moderately strong bar magnet

4. Strong bar magnet

5. Galvanometer (or ammeter)

6. Two connecting wires (preferably with alligator clips)

PROCEDURES

1. Use the wires to connect the ends of the helix coil with few turns to the meter. Record the approximate meter reading when the moderately strong bar magnet is moved at an average speed inside the coil. (If the coil is too small to accommodate the magnet, the magnet may be used to "stroke" the outside of the coil without touching the wires.)

2. Repeat step 1 with the strong bar magnet.

3. Repeat step 2 at high, moderate, and slow speed.

4. Repeat step 2 but with the magnet outside the coil moving at a 90° angle to the wire coils. Record the approximate meter reading at 90°, 45°, and parallel to the wire coils.

5. Repeat step 2 using the coil with few turns and again using the coil with many turns.

ANALYSIS

1. Complete the following data chart:

AMPERE READINGS									
Strength		Speed			Angle			Number of turns	
moderate	strong	slow	moderate	high	90°	45°	0°	few	many

LABORATORY 4-2 (Continued)

2. Which of Faraday's laws is demonstrated by procedure steps 1 and 2?

3. Which of Faraday's laws is demonstrated by procedure step 3?

4. Which of Faraday's laws is demonstrated by procedure step 4?

5. Which of Faraday's laws is demonstrated by procedure step 5?

6. Label the arrows on the following figure to illustrate which indicates the direction of the magnetic field, current, and motion.

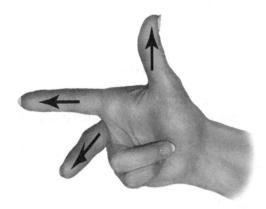

Name _____ Course _____ Date _____

 LABORATORY 7-1 DETERMINING AND CONTROLLING AEC CONFIGURATIONS

PURPOSE

Demonstrate the configuration and correct selection of ion chambers in an automatic exposure control device.

FOR FURTHER REVIEW

Refer to Chapter 7 in the accompanying textbook for further review of this topic.

MATERIALS

1. Energized radiographic unit equipped with an automatic exposure control

2. Image processor

3. 14″× 17″ CR cassette or DR receptor matched to AEC system being tested

4. Abdomen or pelvis phantom

SUGGESTED EXPOSURE FACTORS

400 mA, 80 kVp, 40″ SID, 10:1 or 12:1 Bucky grid, AEC

PROCEDURES

1. Set the tube to 40″ SID, center to the table (if using a CR system, place a 14″ × 17″ CR cassette in the Bucky tray), align to the central ray, and collimate the beam to 14″ × 17″.

2. Select the normal density setting for the AEC system, select the center sensing chamber, expose, and process the image. Mark the image "center chamber."

3. Produce another image by repeating steps 1 and 2 with one of the lateral sensing chambers selected. Mark the image "lateral chamber."

4. Produce another image by repeating steps 1 and 2 with all three sensing chambers selected. Mark the image "all chambers."

RESULTS

1. Review the images with respect to visibility and geometric factors and record each exposure indicator.

ANALYSIS

1. Describe the visual differences, including visibility and geometric factors, in the images.

2. Which image would be the most appropriate for an abdominal survey procedure? Why?

3. Why do the images look similar in appearance even when the exposure indicator values vary?

Name _____ Course _____ Date _____

LABORATORY 7-2 THE EFFECT OF POSITIONING ON AUTOMATIC
EXPOSURE CONTROL

PURPOSE

Demonstrate the effect of positioning errors on the image quality of automatic exposure control radiographs.

FOR FURTHER REVIEW

Refer to Chapter 7 in the accompanying textbook for further review of this topic.

MATERIALS

1. Energized radiographic unit with automatic exposure control

2. Image processor

3. 14″ × 17″ CR cassette or DR receptor matched to AEC system being tested

4. Abdomen or pelvis phantom

SUGGESTED EXPOSURE FACTORS

400 mA, 85 kVp, 40″ SID, 10:1 or 12:1 Bucky grid, AEC

PROCEDURES

1. Set the tube to a 40″ SID, center to the table, position the phantom for a lateral lumbar spine (if using a CR system, place a 14″ × 17″ CR cassette in the Bucky tray), align to the central ray, and collimate to the spine (approximately 6″ × 17″).

2. Select the normal density setting for the AEC system, select the center chamber, expose, and process the image. Mark the image as "baseline."

3. Produce a second image by repeating steps 1 and 2 with the phantom moved 1.5″ posteriorly. Mark the image as "posterior."

4. Produce a third image by repeating steps 1 and 2 with the phantom moved 1.5″ anteriorly. Mark the image as "anterior."

RESULTS

5. Review the images with respect to visibility and geometric factors and record each exposure indicator.

ANALYSIS

1. Which image exhibits the best exposure quality? Why?

2. Why do the images look similar in appearance even when the exposure indicator values vary?

LABORATORY 7-2 (Continued)

3. What caused the exposure indicator value to change between the first and second images?

4. What caused the exposure indicator value to change between the first and third images?

Name _____ Course _____ Date _____

LABORATORY 7-3 THE EFFECT OF COLLIMATION ON AUTOMATIC EXPOSURE CONTROL

PURPOSE

Demonstrate the effects and control of scatter radiation on automatic exposure control radiographs.

FOR FURTHER REVIEW

Refer to Chapter 7 in the accompanying textbook for further review of this topic.

MATERIALS

1. Energized radiographic unit equipped with automatic exposure control

2. Image processor

3. 14″ × 17″ CR cassette or DR receptor matched to the AEC system being tested

4. Abdomen or pelvis phantom

5. Lead masks or lead apron

SUGGESTED EXPOSURE FACTORS

400 mA, 85 kVp, 40″ SID, 10:1 or 12:1 Bucky grid, AEC

PROCEDURES

1. Set the tube to a 40″ SID, center to the table, position the phantom for a lateral lumbar spine (if using a CR system, place a 14″ × 17″ CR cassette in the Bucky tray), align to the central ray, and collimate to a 14″ × 17″ image size.

2. Select the normal density setting for the AEC system, select the center chamber, expose, and process the image. Mark the image "14 × 17."

3. Produce a second image by repeating steps 1 and 2 with the beam collimated to the lumbar spine (6″ × 17″). Mark the image "6 × 17."

4. Produce a third image by repeating steps 1 and 2 with the beam collimated to the lumbar spine (6″ × 17″) with the addition of a lead apron on the table to outline the posterior aspect of the soft tissue. Position the lead apron carefully so as not to overlap the posterior aspect of the phantom. Mark the image "6 × 17 with lead."

RESULTS

1. Review the three images with respect to radiographic exposure indicator value and image contrast.

LABORATORY 7-3 (Continued)

ANALYSIS

1. Which image exhibits the best image contrast? Why?

2. Which image exhibits the worst image contrast? Why?

3. What caused the exposure indicator value to change between the first and second images?

4. What caused the exposure indicator value to change between the second and third images?

UNIT II **Protecting Patients and Personnel**

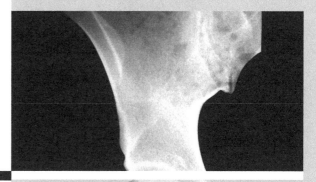

LABORATORY 9-1 USING DOSIMETRY EQUIPMENT

PURPOSE

Use basic ionizing radiation dosimetry equipment.

FOR FURTHER REVIEW

Refer to Chapter 9 in the accompanying textbook for further review of this topic.

MATERIALS

1. Energized radiographic unit
2. Abdomen phantom
3. Ionization Chamber Dosimeter
4. Ring stand

PROCEDURES

1. Position the abdomen phantom on the x-ray table. Use the ring stand to center the dosimeter ionization chamber directly over the sacrum at the point where the beam will enter the phantom.

2. Follow the instructions with the ionization chamber dosimetry equipment to record three exposures to the phantom. Be sure to reset the dosimeter between exposures.

RESULTS

1. Record the three exposures.

ANALYSIS

1. How close to one another were the three exposures?

2. What was the average exposure?

3. If exposures of 65 mR, 62 mR, and 131 mR were recorded   would be advisable to perform three additional exposures. If the second set of exposures were   . mR, 66 mR, and 65 mR, what would you record as the average exposure?

LABORATORY 9-1 (Continued)

4. Why is it advised that the average of three exposures be used for all dosimetry measurements?

5. Why is the roentgen used as the unit of measurement?

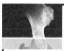 **LABORATORY 10-1** BASIC RADIATION PROTECTION, DETECTION, AND MEASUREMENT

PURPOSE

Introduce commonly used radiation protection techniques and devices and demonstrate their effectiveness in reducing exposure to the patient and operator.

FOR FURTHER REVIEW

Refer to Chapter 10 in the accompanying textbook for further review of this topic.

MATERIALS

1. Energized radiographic unit (assumed to include about 2.5 mm/Al Eq filtration)

2. Abdomen phantom

3. Ionization Chamber Dosimeter

4. Flat contact gonad shields

5. Ring stand

PROCEDURES

1. Become familiar with the common radiation protection devices and techniques as introduced by your instructor.

2. Set up the x-ray tube and phantom as if to do an AP pelvis using a 40″ SID. Raise the phantom with sponges or sheets to create a tunnel large enough to accommodate the dosimeter underneath the phantom.

   A. SOMATIC EXPOSURE—Entrance Skin Exposure (ESE)

      1. Effect of Filtration

         a. Center the dosimeter ionization chamber on the anterior surface of the pelvis. Using a 14″ × 17″ field size, 70 kVp, and 32 mAs, expose and record ESE in mR on Table A. Reset the dosimeter.

         b. Center the dosimeter ionization chamber on the posterior surface of the pelvis. Using a 14″ × 17″ field size, 70 kVp, and 32 mAs, expose and record the exit exposure in mR on Table A. Reset the dosimeter.

         c. Repeat 1a and 1b with 1 mm aluminum added to the primary beam for a total of about 3.5 mm Al.

         d. Repeat 1a and 1b with about 1 mm/Al filtration removed for a total of about 1.5 mm Al.

      2. Effect of kVp

         a. Repeat 1a and 1b but change the technique to 60 kVp and 64 mAs. (This new technique is a result of using the 15 percent rule in order to increase the contrast.)

         b. Repeat 1a and 1b but change the technique to 80 kVp and 16 mAs. (This new technique is a result of using the 15 percent rule in order to decrease the contrast.)

LABORATORY 10-1 (Continued)

B. GONAD EXPOSURE (MALE)

1. Use the ring stand to place the dosimeter ionization chamber at the approximate location of the testes. Collimate the beam so the testes would be included in the beam. Using 70 kVp and 32 mAs, expose and record exposure in mR on Table B. Reset the dosimeter.

2. Repeat B1 using a flat gonad shield placed over the area of the testes.

3. Repeat B1 with the beam collimated to the edge of the area of the testes. Do not use a shield.

4. Repeat B3 using a flat gonad shield placed over the area of the testes.

5. Repeat B1 using a collimated beam that excludes the area of the testes by 5 cm or more. Do not use the shield.

RESULTS

TABLE A

	kVp	mAs	SID	Total Filtration (Al Eq)	ESE (mR)	Exit Exposure (mR)
Effect of Filtration	70	32	40″	2.5 mm Al		
	70	32	40″	3.5 mm Al		
	70	32	40″	1.5 mm Al		
Effect of kVp	60	64	40″	2.5 mm Al		
	80	16	40″	2.5 mm Al		

TABLE B

	Exposure to Testes (mR)	
Beam Collimation	**No Shield**	**Shield**
Include Testes		
Exclude Testes		
Exclude Testes by 5 cm		xxxxxxxxxxxxxxxxx

ANALYSIS

1. Which method(s) investigated reduced the ESEs to the pelvis?

2. Which method had the greatest effect on reducing the ESEs? Why do you think this method is so effective in reducing exposure?

3. Name two other possible methods that could be utilized in reducing the exposure to the patient.

4. List in order the protective methods used in the demonstration according to the gonad exposure received. List the most protective first. Briefly, why do you believe the list is arranged as it is?

5. Why is gonad shielding so important? Why are the male gonads more sensitive to exposure than the female gonads?

Name _____ Course _____ Date _____

 LABORATORY 11-1 HALF-VALUE LAYER DETERMINATION

PURPOSE

Calculate the half-value layer of a given x-ray unit.

FOR FURTHER REVIEW

Refer to Chapter 11 in the accompanying textbook for further review of this topic.

MATERIALS

1. Energized radiographic unit

2. 4 aluminum attenuators (1.0-mm Al sheets)

3. Ionization Chamber Dosimeter

4. Semi-log graph paper

SUGGESTED EXPOSURE FACTORS

100 mAs, 80 kVp, 40″ SID

PROCEDURES

1. Center the dosimeter ionization chamber to the center of the x-ray field. Collimate to a 4″ × 4″ field size.

2. Expose the dosimeter using the suggested exposure factors, record the exposure received by the dosimeter, and reset the dosimeter.

3. Form a shelf below the collimator by loosely taping a 1-mm Al attenuator to the collimator housing. This shelf will be used to hold additional Al attenuators. **NOTE: Make sure the Al attenuator intercepts the entire field of the collimator light. Repeat step 2.**

4. In sequence, add three 1.0-mm Al attenuators to the shelf, repeating step 2 after adding each one.

RESULTS

Dosimeter readings

Filtration	80 kVp
no aluminum added	_____mR
1-mm aluminum added	_____mR
2-mm aluminum added	_____mR
3-mm aluminum added	_____mR
4-mm aluminum added	_____mR

LABORATORY 11-1 (Continued)

ANALYSIS

1. Plot calculated mR values versus total thickness of the Al attenuators added to the x-ray beam, on semi-log graph paper. Draw a straight line through the plotted data points. The thickness of added Al attenuators that reduces the exposure output with 0-mm Al added by one-half is the measured half-value layer. What is the measured half-value layer?

2. According to Table 11-1: Minimum Half Value Layer Requirements for X-ray Systems in the United States in the textbook, what is the minimum HVL for an x-ray tube operating at 80 kVp?

3. What are some of the possible causes for the HVL being less than that recommended? What is/are the practical implication(s) of this situation?

4. What are some of the possible causes for the HVL being excessively large in comparison to the recommended value? What is/are the practical implication(s) of this situation?

5. Define *half-value layer*.

LABORATORY 11-2 EFFECTS OF FILTRATION

PURPOSE

Demonstrate the effect of filtration on x-ray emission.

FOR FURTHER REVIEW

Refer to Chapter 11 in the accompanying textbook for further review of this topic.

MATERIALS

1. Energized radiographic unit
2. Aluminum filters (0.25, 0.5, 1.0, 2.0 mm Al)
3. Ionization Chamber Dosimeter

SUGGESTED EXPOSURE FACTORS

100 mAs, 60 kVp, 40″ SID

PROCEDURES

1. Center the dosimeter ionization chamber to the center of the x-ray field.

2. Direct the central ray perpendicular to the center of the dosimeter ionization chamber and collimate to a 4″ × 4″ field size.

3. Remove all added filtration from the x-ray tube. If this is not possible, the radiographic unit may be used as it is normally filtered. Expose the dosimeter.

4. Record the exposure received by the dosimeter as no aluminum added and reset the dosimeter.

5. Add a 0.25-mm aluminum filter to the primary beam. The aluminum filters may be sequentially taped to the face of the collimator. Expose the dosimeter using the same exposure factors and record the exposure. Reset the dosimeter.

6. Add an additional 0.5-mm aluminum filter and repeat as listed in step 5. Follow the same procedures for 1.0-mm Al and 2.0-mm Al.

7. Reduce the mAs by 50 percent and repeat steps 1 through 8 using 90 kVp.

RESULTS

Dosimeter readings

Filtration	60 kVp	90 kVp
no aluminum added	_____mR	_____mR
0.25-mm aluminum added	_____mR	_____mR
0.5-mm aluminum added	_____mR	_____mR
1.0-mm aluminum added	_____mR	_____mR
2.0-mm aluminum added	_____mR	_____mR

LABORATORY 11-2 (Continued)

ANALYSIS

1. Based on the results obtained, what is the effect of adding filtration on x-ray emission? What is the effect on radiographic exposure?

2. What is the purpose of filtering the radiographic beam?

3. What is the difference among inherent filtration, added filtration, and total filtration?

4. What is the most common filtering material used in diagnostic radiology?

5. What is the total filtration requirement for x-ray tubes that operate at above 70 kVp?

Name _____ Course _____ Date _____

 LABORATORY 12-2 **EFFECT OF mAs, kVp, AND SID ON X-RAY EMISSION**

PURPOSE

Demonstrate the effect of mAs, kVp, and SID on x-ray emission.

FOR FURTHER REVIEW

Refer to Chapter 12 in the accompanying textbook for further review of this topic.

MATERIALS

1. Energized radiographic unit

2. Ionization Chamber Dosimeter

SUGGESTED EXPOSURE FACTORS

100 mA, 0.1 sec, 10 mAs, 50 kVp, 36″ SID

PROCEDURES

1. Place the dosimeter ionization chamber in the center of the x-ray beam.

2. Direct the central ray perpendicular to the center of the ionization chamber and collimate to a 5″ × 5″ field size.

3. Expose the dosimeter, record the results, and reset the dosimeter.

mAs/X-Ray Emission

4. Repeat steps 1 through 3, changing the suggested factors to 20 mAs.

5. Repeat steps 1 through 3, changing the suggested factors to 30 mAs.

kVp/X-Ray Emission

6. Repeat steps 1 through 3, changing the suggested factors to 60 kVp.

7. Repeat steps 1 through 3, changing the suggested factors to 70 kVp.

SID/X-Ray Emission

8. Repeat steps 1 through 3, changing the suggested factors to 56″ SID.

9. Repeat steps 1 through 3, changing the suggested exposure factors to 72″ SID.

LABORATORY 12-2 (Continued)

RESULTS

1. Record the ionization chamber dosimeter readings:

   Initial exposure _____

   mAs/X-ray emission

        20 mAs _____   30 mAs _____

   kVp/X-ray emission

        60 kVp _____   70 kVp _____

   SID/X-ray emission

        56″ SID _____   72″ SID _____

ANALYSIS

mAs/X-Ray Emission

1. What effect does increasing mAs have on the exposure?

2. What is the specific relationship between mAs and x-ray emission?

kVp/X-Ray Emission

3. What effect does increasing kVp have on exposure?

4. What is the specific relationship between kVp and x-ray emission?

SID/X-Ray Emission

5. What effect does increasing SID have on x-ray exposure?

6. What is the specific relationship between SID and x-ray emission?

Name _____ Course _____ Date _____

 LABORATORY 14-1 ESTIMATING PATIENT ENTRANCE SKIN EXPOSURE

PURPOSE

Estimate entrance skin exposure (ESE) for various radiographic projections.

FOR FURTHER READING

Refer to Chapter 14 in the accompanying textbook for further review of this topic.

MATERIALS

1. Energized radiographic unit

2. Ionization Chamber Dosimeter

3. Technique chart

PROCEDURES

1. Obtain a reliable technique chart (ideally one that is used in clinical practice) and, using the techniques from the chart, calculate the ESE values for a 23-cm PA chest, 15-cm lateral skull, 23-cm AP abdomen, 23-cm AP L-Spine, and a 13-cm AP C-Spine according to the following steps.

2. Set the tube SID at the appropriate distance for a PA projection of the chest, place the dosimeter's ionization chamber in the center of the beam, and collimate the beam to the appropriate part size. Set the PA chest exposure factors according to the chart, expose the dosimeter, record the exposure, and reset the dosimeter.

3. Repeat steps 1 and 2 to obtain ESE values for a lateral skull projection, and AP abdomen projection, an AP cervical spine projection, and an AP lumbar spine projection.

4. Determine the thickness of the detector and the distance from the Bucky tray to the tabletop (part image receptor distance) in cm for each projection. Use these figures to determine the source-to-skin distance (SSD) and the source-to-detector distance (SDD).

5. Use the inverse square law to determine the ESE delivered to the body part.

$$\frac{\text{Dosimeter exposure reading (mR)}}{\text{ESE (mR)}} = \frac{\text{SSD}^2}{\text{SDD}^2}$$

Grid Techniques

SSD = SID − (part thickness + part image receptor distance)

SDD = SID − (detector thickness + part image receptor distance)

Tabletop Techniques

SSD = SID − part thickness

SDD = SID − detector thickness

LABORATORY 14-1 (Continued)

RESULTS

1. Record your data below.

	Dosimeter exposure (mR)	SSD (cm)	SDD (cm)	ESE (mR)
PA chest	____	____	____	____
Lateral skull	____	____	____	____
AP abdomen	____	____	____	____
AP C-Spine	____	____	____	____
AP L-Spine	____	____	____	____

ANALYSIS

1. What is the ESE for the five projections?

2. Compare your ESE results with Table 14-2: Medical ESE Values for Selected Radiographic Exams in the textbook.

3. Describe three ways that ESE can be reduced.

4. What correlations can be drawn about ESE and organ dose?

5. ESE decreases as SID increases. What is the new suggested recommendation for SID, and how does it affect patient dose?

Name _____ Course _____ Date _____

 LABORATORY 15-1 BEAM RESTRICTION

PURPOSE

Demonstrate the effects of beam restriction on radiographic image quality.

FOR FURTHER REVIEW

Refer to Chapter 15 in the accompanying textbook for further review of this topic.

MATERIALS

1. Energized radiographic unit

2. Phantom knee

3. 2 water-filled plastic gallon jugs

4. 10″ × 12″ CR cassette or direct capture imaging device with the grid removed

5. Image processor

SUGGESTED EXPOSURE FACTORS

4 mAs, 60 kVp, 40 SID, non-grid

PROCEDURES

1. Position the knee phantom in a PA position for a tabletop, non-grid projection. Place a water-filled jug on each side of the knee to simulate extra tissue. Open the collimators to include as much of the water jugs as possible and make an exposure to obtain the image.

2. Repeat step 1, but collimate the beam closely to include just the knee.

3. Process images.

RESULTS

1. Review the radiographic images with respect to radiographic exposure and scatter exhibited.

ANALYSIS

1. Compare the quality of the two images.

    a.   Which image demonstrates the best image quality? Why?

    b.   Which image demonstrates the lowest exposure? Why?

2. What patient-related factors contribute to the production of scatter radiation?

3. What x-ray-beam-related factors contribute to the production of scatter radiation?

4. Describe two different devices that are used in diagnostic radiology for beam restriction.

UNIT III Creating the Image

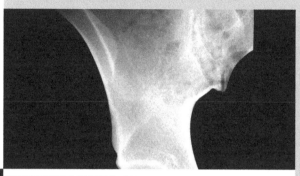

Name _____ Course _____ Date _____

 LABORATORY 16-1 THINKING THREE-DIMENSIONALLY

PURPOSE

Illustrate the importance of multiple projections in perceiving the radiographic image as representation of a three-dimensional object.

FOR FURTHER REVIEW

Refer to Chapter 16 in the accompanying textbook for further review of this topic.

MATERIALS

1. Energized radiographic unit

2. Chest phantom with hollow lung fields is preferred, although a solid chest, abdomen, or pelvis phantom can be substituted

3. 14″ × 17″ image receptor or direct capture imaging device

4. Ionization Chamber Dosimeter

5. Image processor

SUGGESTED EXPOSURE FACTORS

Chest: 6 mAs, 80 kVp, 72″ SID, non-grid Abdomen: 32 mAs, 80 kVp, 40″ SID, 10:1 Bucky grid

PROCEDURES

1. The instructor prepares the phantom by taping several artifacts (keys, hairpins, paper clips, etc.) onto the phantom, at least one each on the surface located anterior, posterior, right lateral, left lateral, and opposite obliques (i.e., right posterior and left anterior surfaces). When a hollow chest phantom can be used, half the artifacts should be inside the chest wall and half outside. Each artifact must be located at a separate superior–inferior location so that no two artifacts will be superimposed on AP, oblique, or lateral radiographs. The prepared phantom is then covered with a patient gown to hide artifact locations from students.

2. Chest phantom: Place the phantom vertically on the tabletop and center it to the image receptor held vertical in a cassette holder. Abdomen/pelvis phantom: Place the phantom recumbent on the table and center it to a loaded image receptor in the Bucky tray or a direct capture imaging device.

3. Direct the central ray perpendicular to the center of the IR, position the phantom for an AP position, and collimate to the part.

4. Expose and process the IR. Label the image by position.

5. Repeat steps 2 through 4 for a left lateral, LPO, and RPO position.

LABORATORY 16-1 (Continued)

RESULTS

1. Number each artifact on all four images (i.e., label the first "artifact #1" on the AP, lateral, and both oblique images; the second "artifact #2" on each image; etc.).

ANALYSIS

1. Give the precise location of each artifact on the phantom. For example, specify location as to anterior, posterior, right or left lateral, RPO, LPO, LAO, RAO surface. For a hollow chest phantom, specify whether the artifact is located inside or outside the chest wall.

2. Give the minimum number of projections necessary to locate each artifact and explain why fewer projections would not define each location.

Name _____ Course _____ Date _____

 LABORATORY 17-1 EFFECT OF SUBJECT ON ATTENUATION AND SCATTER

PURPOSE

Demonstrate the effect of subject thickness on attenuation and scatter of the primary x-ray beam.

FOR FURTHER REVIEW

Refer to Chapter 17 in the accompanying textbook for further review of this topic.

MATERIALS

1. Energized radiographic unit

2. Image processor

3. Abdomen phantom

4. 14 × 17 image receptors

5. 14 × 17 wire mesh test tool

6. Cassette holder

7. Ionization Chamber Dosimeter

8. Densitometer (film/screen)

SUGGESTED EXPOSURE FACTORS

20 mAs, 95 kVp, 40″ SID, non-grid

PROCEDURES

1. Place the abdomen phantom in an AP position on sponges or sheets high enough to create a tunnel of sufficient height to permit the placement of the dosimeter chamber underneath the phantom. Center the phantom to the tabletop with the central ray perpendicular to the level of the iliac crest and collimate to the abdomen. Place the dosimeter detector on the anterior surface of the abdomen at the location of the central ray and expose. Record the ionization chamber dosimeter reading in mR as the entrance exposure.

2. Repeat step 1, but place the dosimeter detector at the posterior surface of the phantom at the location of the central ray. Record the dosimeter reading in mR as the exit exposure.

3. Place the wire mesh test tool on top of a loaded 14″ × 17″ image receptor. Secure both crosswise in a vertical position using a cassette holder as shown in the following figure. Position the cassette holder so that the image receptor is approximately 1 inch from the lateral edge of the phantom and centered to the level of the iliac crest. Using a perpendicular central ray, center the tube to the level of the iliac crest and collimate the beam to the abdomen. The primary beam should not include any portion of the vertical cassette. Expose the phantom using the technique in step 1 and process the image receptor.

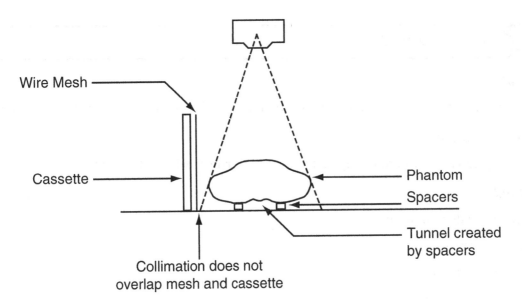

Wire Mesh

Cassette

Phantom

Spacers

Tunnel created
by spacers

Collimation does not
overlap mesh and cassette

4. Position the phantom for a lateral abdomen. Center a perpendicular central ray to the level of the iliac crest and collimate to the phantom, using a 40″ SID. Place the ionization chamber dosimeter detector on the superior lateral surface of the phantom at the location of the central ray. Expose using 5 mAs at 95 kVp. Record the dosimeter reading in mR as the entrance exposure.

5. Repeat step 4, but place the ionization chamber dosimeter detector at the inferior lateral surface of the phantom at the location of the central ray. Record the dosimeter reading in mR as the exit exposure.

6. Place the wire mesh tool on top of a loaded 14 × 17 image receptor. Secure both crosswise in a vertical position using a cassette holder. Position the cassette holder so that the cassette is approximately 1 inch from the posterior surface of the phantom and centered to the level of the iliac crest. Using a perpendicular central ray, center it to the level of the iliac crest and collimate the beam to the phantom. The primary beam should not include the vertical cassette. Expose the phantom using the technique in step 4 and process the image receptor.

7. If using a film/screen receptor, use a densitometer to measure the optical density at the center of the bottom, middle, and top thirds of both radiographs. Record the readings. If using a digital image receptor, record the exposure received by the IR as indicated by the exposure indicator/index recorded in the DICOM information.

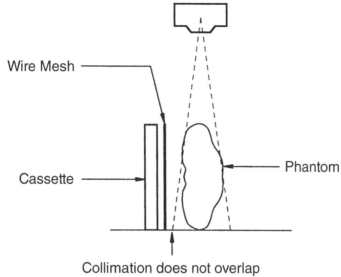

Wire Mesh

Cassette

Phantom

Collimation does not overlap
mesh and cassette

RESULTS

Attenuation

Projection	Part Thickness	Entrance Exposure (mR)	Exit Exposure (mR)
AP Abdomen	_____	_____	_____
Lat Abdomen	_____	_____	_____

Scatter

		OD Image Receptor (film/screen)		
Projection	Part Thickness	Bottom Third	Middle Third	Top Third
AP Abdomen	_____	_____	_____	_____
Lat Abdomen	_____	_____	_____	_____

	OD Image Receptor (digital)	
Projection	Part Thickness	Exposure Indicator
AP Abdomen	_____	_____
Lat Abdomen	_____	_____

ANALYSIS

1. Were the entrance exposures similar or different for the AP and lateral abdomen? Why?

2. Were the exit exposures similar or different for the AP and lateral abdomen? Why?

3. Which radiograph showed the greatest amount of radiographic image receptor exposure? Why?

4. If using film/screen receptor, were you able to demonstrate a difference between the radiographic exposures produced on the bottom, middle, and top thirds of the AP abdomen radiograph? Is so, how would you explain this?

5. If using film/screen receptor, were you able to demonstrate a difference between the radiographic exposures produced on the bottom, middle, and top thirds of the lateral abdomen radiograph? Is so, how would you explain this?

6. What happens to the quality and quantity of the beam as it passes from entrance to exit through the patient? How were these effects demonstrated on the radiographic images you produced as part of this lab?

7. List all the subject-related factors what would have a bearing on attenuation and scatter of the beam.

8. Are there factors besides the subject that affect the attenuation and scatter of the beam? Explain.

9. If the lab was conducted using both film/screen receptors and digital receptors, which imaging system displayed the largest amount of scatter? Why?

Name _____ Course _____ Date _____

 LABORATORY 17-2 THE EFFECT OF PATHOLOGY ON IMAGE QUALITY

PURPOSE

Illustrate the effect of pathology on image quality.

FOR FURTHER REVIEW

Refer to Chapter 17 in the accompanying textbook for further review of this topic.

MATERIALS

Radiographic images demonstrating:

Chest	Abdomen
Congestive heart failure	Ascites
Emphysema	Bowel obstruction
Pleural effusion	
Pneumonia	Extremities/Skull
Tuberculosis	Active osteomyelitis
	Degenerative arthritis
	Osteoporosis
	Paget's disease

ACTIVITIES

1. Based on a review of the radiographic images, which of the images demonstrates an increased attenuation (additive) condition?

2. What causes a pathologic condition to result in an increased attenuation of the x-ray beam?

LABORATORY 17-2 (Continued)

3. Based on a review of the radiographic images, which of the images demonstrates a decreased-attenuation (destructive) condition?

4. What causes a pathologic condition to result in a decreased attenuation of the x-ray beam?

5. Based on a review of the radiographic images, which images required an adjustment from normal technical factors used for the procedure?

6. What technical factor adjustments are recommended for additive conditions? For destructive conditions?

LABORATORY 18-1 GRID COMPARISONS AND CONVERSIONS

PURPOSE

Demonstrate the use of grid conversion factors.

FOR FURTHER REVIEW

Refer to Chapter 18 in the accompanying textbook for further review of this topic.

MATERIALS

1. Energized radiographic unit

2. Image processor

3. 8:1 and 12:1 radiographic grids

4. Abdomen phantom

5. Image receptor

6. Step wedge (penetrometer)

7. Densitometer (if using film/screen image receptors)

SUGGESTED EXPOSURE FACTORS

8 mAs, 70 kVp, 40″ SID, non-grid

PROCEDURES

1. Center the abdomen phantom to the image receptor on the tabletop. Place the step wedge beside the phantom on the image receptor. Direct the central ray perpendicular to the center of the image receptor and collimate to the edges.

2. Use the suggested factors to expose the image receptor, process, and label it "#1." If using a digital imaging receptor, ensure the exposure indicator is within an acceptable range based upon your specific manufacturer's specifications. If the exposure indicator is not in an appropriate range, adjust the mAs and re-expose a new image.

   If using a film/screen receptor, use a densitometer to measure the OD of step 5. If it is not 1.2 ± 0.2, adjust the mAs and re-expose a new image.

3. Repeat step 1 using an 8:1 ratio grid. Expose the image receptor using the appropriate grid conversion factor, process, and label it "#2." If it is not within an acceptable range of exposure as listed above, adjust the mAs and re-expose a new image.

4. Repeat step 1 using a 12:1 ratio grid. Expose the image receptor using the appropriate grid conversion factor, process, and label it "#3." If it is not within an acceptable range of exposure as listed above, adjust the mAs and re-expose a new image.

5. If using a digital imaging system, record the exposure indicators below. If using a film/screen imaging system, use a densitometer to measure the OD (optical density) of step 5 on the step wedge for all the images and record the readings in the results section.

LABORATORY 18-1 (Continued)

RESULTS

1. Review the three images in terms of their exposure.

Exposure indicator or step 5 optical density (OD)

Image #1 _____

Image #2 _____

Image #3 _____

ANALYSIS

1. When is it necessary to use a radiographic grid for an examination?

2. Describe the appearance of images 1, 2, and 3. Which one(s) more closely approximate(s) a quality image? Why?

3. Where were the exposures of the three images the same? If they were not, were the differences significant? Explain.

4. Based on your data, what conclusions can you draw about the effect of grids and grid ratios on conversion factors?

5. What factors or influences contribute to the decrease or increase of image quality in each of the images?

6. Based on the procedure, what is the importance of a radiographic grid?

Name _____ Course _____ Date _____

 LABORATORY 18-2 GRID ERRORS

PURPOSE

Demonstrate the effects of the common errors accompanying the use of radiographic grids.

FOR FURTHER REVIEW

Refer to Chapter 18 in the accompanying textbook for further review of this topic.

MATERIALS

1. Energized radiographic unit

2. Image processor

3. 12:1 80-line/inch linear focused grid

4. Cassettes with image receptor

5. Skull phantom

SUGGESTED EXPOSURE FACTORS

10 mAs, 85 kVp, 40″ SID, 12:1 stationary grid

PROCEDURES

1. Center a 10×12 stationary linear focused grid on a 10×12 image receptor placed crosswise in the center of a radiographic table. Position the phantom skull for a lateral projection, making sure the perpendicular CR is directed to the center of the grid. Expose using the suggested exposure factors.

2. Process the image receptor and label it "exposure #1."

3. Repeat step 1, but move the perpendicular CR approximately 3″ toward the top of the skull so that it is off-center of the grid center line. Open the collimator sufficiently to expose the entire image receptor. Process the image receptor and label it "exposure #2."

4. Repeat step 1, but angle the CR caudally 15° across the grid's center line with it centered to the grid. Adjust the SID to compensate for the angulation and open the collimator sufficiently to expose the entire image receptor. Process the image receptor and label it "exposure #3."

5. Repeat step 1, but elevate the side of the image receptor under the chin 15° from the plane of the table using a positioning sponge. Adjust the phantom skull to maintain its lateral position. Process the image receptor and label it "exposure #4."

6. Repeat step 1, but turn the grid upside down. Make sure the CR is centered to the grid. Process the image receptor and label it "exposure #5."

7. Repeat step 1, but use a 50″ SID. Process the image receptor and label it "exposure #6."

8. Repeat step 1, but use a 30″ SID. Process the image receptor and label it "exposure #7."

LABORATORY 18–2 (Continued)

RESULTS

1. Using image 1 as the standard for comparison, review the six images with respect to image quality.

ANALYSIS

1. Describe images 2 through 7 with respect to their image quality.

2. Which grid error(s) had the worst effect on the image quality? Explain the reason for this occurrence.

3. Which grid error(s) had the least effect on the image quality? Explain the reason for this occurrence.

4. Would you expect the results to be more or less severe with a lower-ratio grid? Justify your answer.

5. Based on the results of the experiment, state at least four rules that should be followed when using linear grids.

LABORATORY 18-3 THE MOIRE EFFECT WHEN UTILIZING COMPUTED RADIOGRAPHIC SYSTEMS

PURPOSE

To demonstrate the appearance and cause of a moire effect grid artifact when utilizing CR imaging systems.

FOR FURTHER REVIEW

Refer to Chapter 18 in the accompanying textbook for further review of this topic.

MATERIALS

1. Energized radiographic unit

2. Two 10 × 12 CR cassettes

3. Skull phantom

4. 8:1 ratio 10 × 12 stationary linear (LD) grid with a frequency higher than 178 lines/inch

5. 8:1 ratio 10 × 12 stationary linear (LD) grid with a frequency lower than 178 lines/inch

SUGGESTED EXPOSURE FACTORS

85 kVp, 10 mAs, 40″ SID

PROCEDURES

1. Position the skull for a lateral skull using a 10 × 12 image receptor and the 8:1 ratio grid with a frequency higher than 178 lines/inch crosswise (landscape) on the tabletop. Center and collimate the beam to the cassette. Exposure the receptor and process it using a lateral skull algorithm, marking the image "#1,178 crosswise."

2. Repeat step 1 using the 8:1 ratio grid with a frequency lower than 178 lines/inch. Expose the receptor and process it using a lateral skull algorithm, marking the image "#2,178 crosswise."

3. Repeat step 1, placing the image receptor and grid in a vertical (portrait) position. Expose and process it using a lateral skull algorithm, marking the image "#3,178 vertical."

4. Repeat step 2, placing the receptor and grid in a vertical (portrait) position, Expose and process it using a lateral skull algorithm, marking the image "#4,178 vertical."

RESULTS

1. Visually review and compare the four skull images with regard to image quality.

2. Record the exposure indicator for each image.

LABORATORY 18-3 (Continued)

ANALYSIS

1. Was there a difference in the appearance of grid lines on the four images? If so, is the difference significant?

2. Which grid had the worst effect on image quality? Explain the reason for this occurrence.

3. Does placing the grid in a vertical (portrait) versus crosswise (landscape) position change the appearance of the image in terms of grid artifact? Why or why not?

UNIT IV **Digital Radiography Introduction**

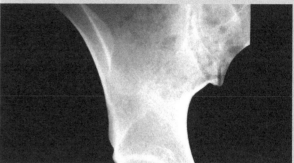

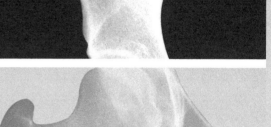

Name _____ Course _____ Date _____

 LABORATORY 20-2 CONTROLLING AND EVALUATING DIGITAL IMAGES

PURPOSE

Explain the function of digital image window level and width controls.

FOR FURTHER REVIEW

Refer to Chapter 20 in the accompanying textbook for further review of this topic.

MATERIALS

1. Energized radiographic unit

2. CR or DR imaging receptor

3. Image processor

4. Forearm phantom

SUGGESTED EXPOSURE FACTORS

60 kVp, 5 mAs, 40″ SID non-grid

PROCEDURE

1. Using a digital image receptor, produce a diagnostic-quality image of a phantom body part.

2. Expose the forearm image and process the image using the correct algorithm for a forearm image. Use only the window level control to make the image completely light. Record this number. Carefully observe the effect on the demonstration of various structures as the window level is slowly increased to complete darkness. Record this number. Bring the window level back to the original number. Watch the monitor closely while the window level is very slowly increased. Record the number when the first visible change is observed.

3. Use only the window width control to make the image completely light. Record this number. Carefully observe the effect on the demonstration of various structures as the window width is slowly increased to complete darkness. Record this number. Bring the window width back to the original number. Watch the monitor closely while the window width is very slowly increased. Record the number when the first visible change is observed.

RESULTS

1. Record the window level and width numbers as indicated in the preceding procedures.

2. Subtract the window level number for the light image from the dark image and record the result as the range (R). Subtract the window level number for the light image from the original diagnostic-quality image and record the result as the diagnostic level (D). Use the formula D/R × 100 to determine the percentage of window level that produced the diagnostic image.

3. Repeat this process for the window width numbers.

LABORATORY 20-2 (Continued)

ANALYSIS

1. What visible image quality factor is changing as the window level is varied?

2. What visible image quality factor is changing as the window width is varied?

3. What percentage change was required to see a brightness change?

4. What percentage change was required to see a contrast change?

5. What percent of the total available range of contrast produced the diagnostic-quality image?

Name _____ Course _____ Date _____

 LABORATORY 20-3 CR/DR EXPOSURE FACTOR SELECTION

PURPOSE

Investigate the exposure latitude characteristics of a given CR or DR system.

FOR FURTHER REVIEW

Refer to Chapter 20 in the accompanying textbook for further review of this topic.

MATERIALS

1. Energized radiographic unit

2. CR or DR image receptors

3. Image processor

4. Skull phantom

SUGGESTED EXPOSURE FACTORS

85 kVp, 10 mAs, 40″ SID, 10:1 or 12:1 grid

PROCEDURE A: EXPOSURE COMPENSATION LIMITS FOR MAS

1. Using a CR or DR image receptor, produce a diagnostic-quality image of a lateral skull. Process the image and label it "mAs baseline."

2. Maintaining all other factors above, produce four additional images changing only the mAs as follows:

   a. Decrease the mAs by ¼

   b. Decrease the mAs by ½

   c. Increase the mAs × 2

   d. Increase the mAs × 4

3. Process each image and label each image according to the change in mAs.

PROCEDURE B: EXPOSURE COMPENSATION LIMITS FOR KVP

1. Using a CR or DR image receptor, produce a diagnostic-quality image of a lateral skull. Process the image and label it "kVp baseline."

2. Maintaining all other factors above, produce four additional images changing only the kVp as follows:

   a. Decrease the kVp by 30 percent

   b. Decrease the kVp by 15 percent

   c. Increase the kVp by 15 percent

   d. Increase the kVp by 30 percent

3. Process each image and label each image according to the change in kVp.

LABORATORY 20-3 (Continued)

RESULTS

Review the images produced in Procedures A and B in respect to image quality.

ANALYSIS

1. Considering the set of images produced in Procedures A and B, which would you be willing to submit for diagnosis?

2. What is your assessment of the CR/DR compensation range for insufficient and excessive mAs?

3. What is your assessment of the CR/DR compensation range for insufficient and excessive kVp?

4. In reviewing the images in Procedures A and B, are you able to detect a difference in the level of noise present in the images? How would you account for this?

5. What recommendations can you make for this CR/DR system for setting technical factors? Be sure you include both high and low ranges as well as specify how close factors must be to an appropriate manual exposure technique to produce acceptable-quality images.

LABORATORY 21-1 COMPUTED RADIOGRAPHIC PROCESSING ERRORS

PURPOSE

Demonstrate the effect of common errors in obtaining and processing computed radiographic images.

FOR FURTHER REVIEW

Refer to Chapter 21 in the accompanying textbook for further review of this topic.

MATERIALS

1. Energized radiographic unit

2. 8″ × 10″ or 10″ × 12″ CR image receptors

3. Wrist phantom

4. Image processor

SUGGESTED EXPOSURE FACTORS

50 kVp, 3 mAs, non-grid tabletop, 40″ SID

PROCEDURES

1. Erase all CR receptors before beginning this laboratory to ensure they are clean.

2. Place a CR receptor on top of a radiographic table. Center the wrist phantom to the middle of the receptor and center the CR for a proper wrist image. Collimate the beam so that there is at least a 25-inch collimated border on all four sides of the image.

3. Place a second CR receptor on the tabletop approximately 1 foot from the cassette being used to image the wrist. This receptor should remain on the tabletop for all four exposures, but NOT be exposed to the primary x-ray beam. It will be used to evaluate the CR system's sensitivity to scatter radiation.

4. Expose the wrist image and process the image using the correct algorithm for a PA wrist image. Label this image "#1, baseline image." Evaluate this image and record the exposure index. Adjust the technical exposure factors, if necessary, to obtain an image within the acceptable exposure indicator range.

5. Repeat step 1, but process the image using an abdomen algorithm. Label this image "#2, histogram error." Evaluate the image and record the exposure index.

6. Repeat step 1, placing the wrist phantom off-center to the left of the cassette. Collimate the beam so that there is at least a 2-inch collimated border on all four sides of the image.

7. Expose the wrist image and process the image using the correct algorithm for a PA wrist image. Label this image "#3, off-center error." Evaluate the image and record the exposure index.

8. Repeat step 1, placing the wrist phantom off-center to the left of the receptor. Adjust the collimator so that the radiation field extends beyond the left side, top, and bottom of the cassette (only the right side should have a crisp collimated border).

LABORATORY 21-1 (Continued)

9. Expose the wrist image and process the image using the correct algorithm for a PA wrist image. Label this image "#4, collimator edge identification error." Evaluate the image and record the exposure index.

10. Process the CR image receptor left on the tabletop for the three exposures using the algorithm for a PA wrist image. Mark this image as "#5, CR scatter sensitivity." Evaluate the image and record the exposure index.

RESULTS

1. Compare image 1 and image 2.

    a. What effect is seen as a result of the histogram error?

    b. What is the basis for the difference in the two images?

    c. Are both images of diagnostic quality?

    d. Are the exposure indices different? Why or why not?

2. Compare image 1 and image 3.

    a. What effect is seen as a result of the off-center positioning error?

    b. What is the basis for the difference in the two images?

    c. Are both images of diagnostic quality?

    d. Are the exposure indices different? Why or why not?

3. Compare image 1 and image 4.

    a. What effect is seen as a result of the collimator edge index error?

    b. What is the basis for the difference in the two images?

    c. Are both images of diagnostic quality?

    d. Are the exposure indices different? Why or why not?

4. What effect is seen as a result of the scatter radiation on image 5?

    a. Why is this information important in a clinical imaging environment?

5. Of the four errors made in utilizing the CR system, which error most greatly affected the image quality?

UNIT V   Analyzing the Image

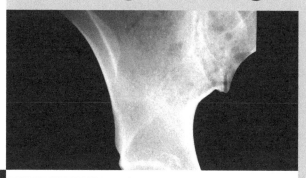

Name _____ Course _____ Date _____

 LABORATORY 25-1 EVALUATING ACCEPTANCE LIMITS

PURPOSE

Determine the approximate diagnostic image quality acceptance limits for screen/film receptors and digital radiographic systems.

FOR FURTHER REVIEW

Refer to Chapter 25 in the accompanying textbook for further review of this topic.

MATERIALS

1. Energized radiographic unit

2. 14″ × 17″ screen/film image receptors 400 RS

3. 14″ × 17″ CR image receptor or a DR unit

4. Abdomen or pelvis phantom

5. Automatic film processor

6. CR image processor

SUGGESTED EXPOSURE FACTORS

First exposure: 80 kVp, 2.5 mAs, 40″ SID, grid

PROCEDURES

1. Position the abdomen phantom for an AP projection using a screen/film IR. Center and collimate the beam to the IR. Expose and process the image.

2. Repeat step 1 to produce a series of phantom images by increasing the exposure by 2 × mAs increments (5 mAs, 10 mAs, 20 mAs, 40 mAs, 80 mAs, 160 mAs). Process the images and clearly number with the corresponding mAs values.

3. Repeat steps 1 and 2 using a digital imaging receptor. Process the images using an AP abdomen algorithm and clearly number with the corresponding mAs values.

RESULTS

1. Arrange the entire screen/film series on viewboxes in order of increasing mAs. If the digital images are printed to film, also arrange them on viewboxes in order of increasing mAs. If the digital images are viewed on a monitor, sequence the images for viewing from lowest mAs to highest mAs.

2. Survey as many radiologists, radiographers, and students as possible. Ask each professional to record only those images that are unacceptable for diagnosis in each set of images. The goal is to determine which images from each set could be submitted for diagnosis, not which is the best image.

LABORATORY 25-1 (Continued)

3. Create two subsets of histogram graphs (x-axis = mAs value, y-axis = number of respondents submitting image for diagnosis) by drawing vertical bars to indicate how many persons said they would submit each image for diagnosis. The subset should be created as follows:

   a. Screen/film images
       i. Radiologists
      ii. Radiographers
     iii. Students

   b. Digital images
       i. Radiologists
      ii. Radiographers
     iii. Students

ANALYSIS

1. Compare the histograms for each subset and discuss why the groups are similar or different.

2. Compare the histograms for the same population by comparing screen/film images to digital images, and discuss the differences and similarities.

3. Compare your personal opinion of the images in both sets to the results you obtained for each group. Explain the possible reasons for all differences.

4. How do the acceptable ranges vary from screen/film to digital receptors?

5. According to your data, which system exhibits the widest latitude? Explain your answer.

6. Knowledge of the diagnostic process is necessary for the radiographer to diagnose and treat the image. List the four major steps in the diagnostic process-solving strategy.

7. List the advantages and disadvantages of utilizing an image receptor with a wide latitude.

LABORATORY 26-1 THE EFFECT OF mAs ON IR EXPOSURE

PURPOSE

Demonstrate the effect of mAs on image IR exposure.

FOR FURTHER REVIEW

Refer to Chapter 26 in the accompanying textbook for further review of this topic.

MATERIALS

1. Energized radiographic unit

2. 10″ × 12″ CR cassette or direct capture imaging device with the grid removed

3. Wrist phantom

4. Step wedge

5. Image processor

SUGGESTED EXPOSURE FACTORS

First exposure: 50 kVp, 2.0 mAs, 40″ SID, non-grid

PROCEDURES

Part A

1. Place a 10″ × 12″ image receptor (IR) crosswise on top of the radiographic table. Using lead masks, divide into thirds in a crosswise fashion to obtain three exposures on one IR.

2. Center the wrist phantom and step wedge on the unmasked portion. Label this image "A." Center and collimate the beam to the unmasked portion of the IR. Expose the IR.

3. Rearrange the masks and place the phantom in the middle section of the IR. Center and collimate the beam to the unmasked portion of the IR. Expose using 50 kVp, 4 mAs, 40″ SID.

4. Rearrange the masks and place the phantom in the final third of the IR. Center and collimate the beam to the unmasked portion of the IR. Expose the cassette using 50 kVp, 8 mAs, 40″ SID. Process the image.

5. Record the exposure received by the IR as indicated by the exposure indicator/index recorded in the DICOM information.

Part B (Only if you have radiographic unit that allows the operator to choose mA and time separately)

1. Place a 10″ × 12″ IR crosswise on top of the radiographic table. Using lead masks, divide the IR into thirds in a crosswise fashion to obtain three exposures on one IR.

2. Center the wrist phantom and step wedge on the unmasked portion. Label this image "B." Center and collimate the beam to the unmasked portion of the IR. Expose using 50 kVp, 50 mA, 1/10 sec, and 40″ SID.

LABORATORY 26-1 (Continued)

3. Rearrange the masks and place the phantom in the middle section of the IR. Center and collimate the beam to the unmasked portion of the IR. Expose using 50 kVp, 100 mA, 1/20 sec, 40″ SID.

4. Rearrange the masks and place the phantom in the final third of the IR. Center and collimate the beam to the unmasked portion of the IR. Expose using 50 kVp, 200 mA, 1/40 sec, 40″ SID. Process the image.

5. Record the exposure received by the IR as indicated by the exposure indicator/index recorded in the DICOM information.

RESULTS

Image A	2.0 mAs	4 mAs	8 mAs
OD step 6			

Image B	50 mAs, 1/10 sec	100 mA, 1/20 sec	200 mA, 1/40 sec
OD step 6			

ANALYSIS

1. What is the effect observed on the radiographic IR exposure of each of the three images in Part A as the mAs is increased?

2. What is the physical basis for the occurrence of these changes?

3. Do these results prove the theory proposed in Chapter 26 of the textbook? Why or why not?

4. Review the EI values of each of the three images in Part B. What is the effect observed on the IR exposure?

5. What is the physical basis for this occurrence?

6. What law is supported or not supported by the results Part B?

LABORATORY 26-2 THE EFFECT OF kVp ON IR EXPOSURE—
THE 15 PERCENT RULE

PURPOSE

Demonstrate the effects of kilovoltage on IR exposure and the control of IR exposure by changing kVp and mAs utilizing the 15 percent rule.

FOR FURTHER REVIEW

Refer to Chapter 26 in the accompanying textbook for further review of this topic.

MATERIALS

1. Energized radiographic unit
2. Image processor
3. 14″ × 17″ image receptor
4. Knee phantom
5. Step wedge

SUGGESTED EXPOSURE FACTORS

400 RS, see procedure for mA, sec, and kVp, 40″ SID, non-grid

PROCEDURES

A. kVp versus Image Exposure

1. Place a 14″ × 17″ image receptor (IR) crosswise on top of the radiographic table. Using lead masks, divide the IR into thirds in a crosswise fashion for three exposures on one receptor.
2. Center the phantom knee and step wedge on the unmasked portion. Label the image "A," center the central ray, and collimate the beam to the unmasked portion of the receptor. Make an exposure at 75 kVp, 2 mAs, and 40" SID.
3. Rearrange the masks to reveal the middle third of the IR and repeat step 2. Change the kVp to 65 and expose. Rearrange the masks to reveal the final third of the IR and repeat step 2. Change the kVp to 86 and expose.
4. Process image A.
5. Record the exposure received by the IR as indicated by the exposure indicator (EI) recorded in the DICOM information.

B. 15 Percent Rule for Image Exposure Control

1. Place a 14″ × 17″ IR crosswise on top of the radiographic table. Using lead masks, divide the IR into thirds in a crosswise fashion for three exposures on one image receptor.
2. Center the phantom knee and step wedge on the unmasked portion. Label the receptor, center the central ray, and collimate the beam to the unmasked portion of the receptor. Make an exposure at 75 kVp, 2 mAs, and 40″ SID.
3. Rearrange the masks to reveal the middle third of the cassette and repeat step 2. Decrease the kVp to 65 and, using the 15 percent rule, calculate the mAs to be used with the new kVp and expose the receptor.

LABORATORY 26-2 (Continued)

4. Rearrange the masks to reveal the final third of the IR and repeat step 2. Increase the kVp to 86 and, using the 15 percent rule, calculate the mAs to be used with the new kVp and expose the receptor.

5. Process image B.

6. Record the exposure received by the IR as indicated by the exposure indicator (EI) recorded in the DICOM information.

RESULTS

OD step 6

	75 kV	65 kV	86 kV
Image A	_____	_____	_____
Image B	_____	_____	_____

ANALYSIS

1. Discuss the image receptor exposure of the three images in procedure A using both visual and quantitative data.

2. Discuss the image receptor exposure of the three images in procedure B using both visual and quantitative data.

3. How do the visual and quantitative results in procedure B compare with the images obtained with similar kVp used in procedure A? Explain.

4. What is the theory behind the results in procedure B? Do your results support the theory? Explain.

5. What observations can you make about the contrast of the three images in procedure B? In procedure A?

6. Why does kVp not effect contrast in a digital image?

LABORATORY 26-3 DETERMINING ADEQUATE PENETRATION

PURPOSE

Demonstrate the effects of x-ray penetration in regard to adequate demonstration of the visibility of the object imaged using both screen/film and CR/digital radiographic receptors.

FOR FURTHER REVIEW

Refer to Chapter 26 in the accompanying textbook for further review of this topic.

MATERIALS

1. Energized radiographic unit

2. Skull phantom

3. Image processor

4. 10″ × 12″ screen/film image receptor

5. 10″ × 12″ CR image receptor

6. Densitometer

SUGGESTED EXPOSURE FACTORS

Initial exposure: 80 kVp, 10 mAs, 40″ SID, 8:1 Bucky grid

PROCEDURES

1. Place a film/screen image receptor (IR) in the Bucky tray and position the phantom on the tabletop for a lateral skull, with the central ray centered to the sella turcica. Collimate to the IR size, and expose and process the image. Label as #1.

2. Repeat step 1, but reduce the kVp to 40 and increase the mAs to 100. Expose and process the image. Label as #2.

3. Repeat step 2, but increase the mAs to 400. Expose and process the image. Label as #3.

4. Repeat steps 1, 2, and 3 using CR cassettes and label the images #4, #5, and #6.

RESULTS

1. Review the three screen/film images side by side, comparing the images for visibility of the petrous portion of the temporal bone and for adequate image receptor exposure.

2. If possible, print the three CR images to film and review them side by side, comparing the images for visibility of the petrous portion of the temporal bone and for adequate image receptor exposure. If this is not possible, view the images on a high-resolution monitor to make the visual comparison.

LABORATORY 26-3 (Continued)

3. If using a film/screen receptor, use a densitometer to measure the optical density in the parietal bone region of the skull and in the petrous portion of the skull for all three images. If using a digital image receptor, record the exposure received by the IR as indicated by the exposure indicator/index recorded in the DICOM information.

Image	OD Parietal Bone	OD Petrous Portion	Within Useful OD Range?
1			
2			
3			
4			
5			
6			

ANALYSIS

1. Do the OD readings on any of the images fall within the useful OD range?

2. Which images demonstrate the achievement of satisfactory IR exposure and optimal visibility of the petrous portion of the temporal bone? Why?

3. Would satisfactory IR exposure of the area of interest be achieved if the mAs was increased to 800 or 1,000? Explain.

4. Describe differences between the screen/film and CR images. Explain the rationale for these differences.

LABORATORY 26-4 THE EFFECT OF DISTANCE ON IR EXPOSURE—THE
EXPOSURE MAINTENANCE FORMULA

PURPOSE

Demonstrate the effect of SID on IR exposure and the use of the exposure maintenance formula to control IR exposure.

FOR FURTHER REVIEW

Refer to Chapter 26 in the accompanying textbook for further review of this topic.

MATERIALS

1. Energized radiographic unit
2. Image processor
3. 14″ × 17″ image receptors
4. Knee phantom
5. Step wedge (penetrometer)
6. Densitometer

SUGGESTED EXPOSURE FACTORS

See procedure for mA, sec, and kVp, 40″ SID, non-grid

PROCEDURES

Distance and IR Exposure

1. Place a 14″ × 17″ IR crosswise on top of the radiographic table. Using lead masks, divide the IR into thirds in a crosswise fashion for three exposures on one image receptor.

2. Center the knee phantom and step wedge on the unmasked portion. Label the image "A," center the central ray, and collimate the beam to the unmasked portion of the image. Select 70 kVp, 2 mAs, and 40″ SID, and expose the image receptor.

3. Rearrange the masks to reveal the middle third of the IR and repeat step 2. Adjust the SID to 60″ and expose the image receptor.

4. Rearrange the masks to reveal the final third of the IR and repeat step 2. Adjust the SID to 20″, expose the image receptor, and process it.

5. If using a film/screen receptor, use a densitometer to measure and record the OD of step 6 of the step wedge. If using a digital image receptor, record the exposure received by the IR as indicated by the exposure indicator/index recorded in the DICOM information.

Exposure Maintenance Formula

1. Place a 14″ × 17″ IR crosswise on top of the radiographic table. Using lead masks, divide the IR into thirds in a crosswise fashion for three exposures on one image receptor.

2. Center the knee phantom and step wedge on unmasked portion. Label the image "B," center the central ray, and collimate the beam to the unmasked portion of the image receptor. Select 70 kVp, 2 mAs, and 40″ SID, and expose the image receptor.

Chapter 26   Image Receptor Exposure   **123**

LABORATORY 26-4 (Continued)

3. Rearrange the masks to reveal the middle third of the IR and repeat step 2. Increase the SID to 60″ and, using the exposure maintenance formula, calculate the mAs to be used with the new distance to maintain the image receptor exposure and expose the image receptor.

4. Rearrange the masks to reveal the final third of the IR and repeat step 2. Decrease the SID to 20″ and, using the exposure maintenance formula, calculate the mAs to be used with the new distance, expose, and process the image receptor.

5. If using a film/screen receptor, use a densitometer to measure and record the OD of step 6 of the step wedge. If using a digital image receptor, record the exposure received by the IR as indicated by the exposure indicator/index recorded in the DICOM information.

RESULTS

	OD step 6		
	40″	60″	20″
Image A	_____	_____	_____
Image B	_____	_____	_____

ANALYSIS

1. As the SID is increased, what effect is seen in the IR exposure of each of the three images on image A?

2. What is the physical basis for the changes seen on image A?

3. What effect does the manipulation of mAs have on IR exposure (image B)?

4. What is the physical basis for the results demonstrated on image B?

5. Briefly describe the practical importance of the mAs/distance relationships as seen on image B.

Name _____ Course _____ Date _____

PURPOSE

Demonstrate the effect of different relative speed combinations on image receptor exposure.

FOR FURTHER REVIEW

Refer to Chapter 26 in the accompanying textbook for further review of this topic.

MATERIALS

1. Energized radiographic unit

2. Image processor

3. Various speed image receptors

4. Knee phantom

5. Densitometer

6. Step wedge (penetrometer)

SUGGESTED EXPOSURE FACTORS

See procedure for RS, 100 mA, 0.05 sec, 60 kVp, 40″ SID, non-grid

PROCEDURES

1. Produce an image of the knee phantom and step wedge with each of the following RS combinations that are available. Use the same exposure factors for each, with the central ray centered and perpendicular to the knee, the step wedge parallel to the knee, and the beam collimated to the IR size.

   a. Detail (100 RS)   c. Regular (400 RS)

   b. Medium (250 RS)   d. Fast (800 RS)

2. Use a densitometer to measure and record the OD of the middle step (step 6) of each of the four step wedge images.

RESULTS

                                OD step 6

   Detail   _____

   Medium   _____

   Regular   _____

   Fast   _____

LABORATORY 26-5 (Continued)

ANALYSIS

1. What inferences can be made from the differences in the image receptor exposures on each of the images?

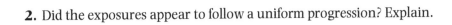

2. Did the exposures appear to follow a uniform progression? Explain.

3. What physical factors dictate the speed (sensitivity) of an intensifying screen?

4. How do screen manufacturers vary the speed of intensifying screens during their construction?

5. What is the purpose of having such a wide variety of screen speeds available?

LABORATORY 26-6 THE EFFECT OF TISSUE DENSITY AND CONTRAST ON IR EXPOSURE

PURPOSE

Demonstrate the effect of different tissue densities and contrast on IR Exposure.

FOR FURTHER REVIEW

Refer to Chapter 26 in the accompanying textbook for further review of this topic.

MATERIALS

1. Energized radiographic unit
2. Image processor
3. 8″ × 10″ image receptor
4. Shallow container (about 3″ to 4″ deep)
5. Ice cubes
6. 35-mm film canister
7. Super ball 1″ diameter
8. Barium solution

SUGGESTED EXPOSURE FACTORS

See procedure for mAs and kVp, 40″ SID, non-grid

PROCEDURES

NOTE: The images produced for this laboratory are also used for Laboratory 29-3, The Effect of Tissue Density and Subject Contrast on Image Contrast.

Tissue Density and IR Exposure

1. Fill the container with enough ice cubes to form a single layer. Add water to equal the height of the ice cubes.

2. Mask a IR in half, center the container to the unmasked portion, collimate, label image #1, and expose at 45 kVp, 1.00 mAs, and 40″ SID.

3. Add water to increase the depth to 2″ in the container. Use the other half of the IR to repeat steps 2 and 3 and process the image.

Tissue Contrast and IR Exposure

1. Place a super ball in an empty 35-mm film canister. Fill the canister with water and replace the cap. Fill the shallow container with water to a depth of 3″ and add the canister.

2. Mask a IR in quarters, center the container to an unmasked portion, collimate, label image #2, and expose at 60 kVp, 6 mAs, and 40″ SID.

3. Remove the water from the canister and replace the super ball and cap. Place the canister in the shallow container, change the mask, and repeat step 2.

4. Fill the canister with a liquid barium suspension, replace the super ball and the cap to the canister. Place the film canister in the shallow container. Change the mask and repeat step 2.

5. Remove the barium from the canister, rinse well with water, replace the super ball in the empty canister, and replace the cap. Change the mask and center the canister directly to an unmasked quarter of the IR (do not place the film canister in the shallow container). Center, collimate, and expose using 60 kVp, 1 mAs, and 40″ SID.

6. Process the image.

RESULTS

1. Review both sets of images for IR exposures.

ANALYSIS

1. What caused the different image receptor exposures seen in image #1?

2. Why are fewer image receptor exposures seen in exposure two on image #1?

3. Which image demonstrates the greatest number of image receptor exposures on image #2? Why?

4. Which image demonstrates the least number of image receptor exposures on image #2? Why?

5. Assuming the super ball is a solid tumor, which of the first three images demonstrates its tissue density the best? Why?

Name _____ Course _____ Date _____

 LABORATORY 27-1 THE EFFECT OF kVp ON IMAGE CONTRAST

PURPOSE

Demonstrate the effects of kVp on image contrast.

FOR FURTHER REVIEW

Refer to Chapter 27 in the accompanying textbook for further review of this topic.

MATERIALS

1. Energized radiographic unit

2. Image processor

3. CR image receptor or DR unit

4. 10 × 12 film screen image receptor

5. Step wedge

6. Skull phantom

7. Densitometer (if using film/screen image receptors)

SUGGESTED EXPOSURE FACTORS

100 mA, 20 sec, 60 kVp, 40″ SID, 8:1 Bucky grid

PROCEDURES

1. Use a 10″ × 12″ image receptor (IR) to produce a lateral skull with a step wedge placed adjacent to it.

2. If using film/screen, use a densitometer to record the OD of steps 4, 5, and 6 of the step wedge. If the OD of step 5 is not 1.2 ± 0.2, adjust the mAs and re-expose.

3. If using a digital imaging receptor, ensure the exposure indicator (EI) is within an acceptable range based upon your specific manufacturer's specifications. If the exposure indicator is not in an appropriate range, adjust the mAs and re-expose a new image.

4. Repeat steps 1 and 2 using 80 kVp, 10 mAs, and 40″ SID.

5. Repeat steps 1 and 2 using 96 kVp, 5.0 mAs, and 40″ SID.

RESULTS

1. Record the OD of steps 4, 5, and 6 below.

2. Calculate the image contrast of each image by subtracting the OD of step 6 from the OD of step 4.

kVp	Step Wedge Optical Density			Contrast
	Step 4	Step 5	Step 6	Step 4 through Step 6
60	_____	_____	_____	_____
80	_____	_____	_____	_____
96	_____	_____	_____	_____

LABORATORY 27-1 (Continued)

ANALYSIS

1. Compare the overall image receptor exposure of each image individually and then compare the overall exposures between the images. Describe your observations. Do your data support your findings? Explain.

2. Describe the observed differences in the contrast between the three images. Explain the reason for the results. Do your data support your observations? Explain.

3. Why do you think it would be advantageous to be able to change the contrast of an image?

4. Define *image contrast.*

5. Explain the difference between long-scale contrast and short-scale contrast.

LABORATORY 27-2 THE EFFECT OF TISSUE DENSITY AND CONTRAST ON IMAGE CONTRAST

PURPOSE

Demonstrate the effect of different tissue densities and subject contrast on image contrast.

FOR FURTHER REVIEW

Refer to Chapter 27 in the accompanying textbook for further review of this topic.

MATERIALS

1. Energized radiographic unit

2. Image processor

3. 8″ × 10″ image receptors

4. Shallow container (about 3″ to 4″ deep)

5. Ice cubes

6. 35-mm film canister

7. Super ball 1″ diameter size

8. Barium solution

SUGGESTED EXPOSURE FACTORS

See procedure for mAs and kVp, 40″ SID, non-grid

PROCEDURES

Use the images produced for Laboratory 26-6, The Effect of Tissue Density and Contrast on IR Exposure. If Laboratory 26-6 was not done previously, use the procedures section from that laboratory to produce the image for this laboratory.

RESULTS

1. Review the exposures on both images for image contrast.

ANALYSIS

1. What caused the different contrast ranges seen in image 1?

2. Why was the contrast reduced in the second exposure on image 1?

3. Which exposure demonstrates the greatest contrast on image 2? Why?

4. Which exposure demonstrates the least contrast on image 2? Why?

5. Assuming the super ball is a solid tumor, which of the first three images demonstrates its contrast the best? Why?

LABORATORY 27-3 THE EFFECT OF EXPOSURE LATITUDE
ON IMAGE CONTRAST

PURPOSE

Demonstrate how exposure latitude affects image contrast.

FOR FURTHER REVIEW

Refer to Chapter 27 in the accompanying textbook for further review of this topic.

MATERIALS

1. Energized radiographic unit

2. Image processor

3. 10″ × 12″ image receptors

4. Hand phantom

SUGGESTED EXPOSURE FACTORS

See procedure for mAs and kVp, 40″ SID, non-grid

PROCEDURES

1. Mask a image receptor in half crosswise and center it to the top of the radiographic table. Center the hand phantom to the unmasked portion of the IR, label it "exposure #1," collimate to the image size, and expose using 45 kVp and 10 mAs.

2. Repeat step 1, labeling it "exposure #2," expose using 55 kVp and 10 mAs, and process the image receptor.

3. Repeat steps 1 and 2. Label the first half "exposure #3" and expose using 73 kVp and 2.5 mAs. Label the second half "exposure #4" and expose using 83 kVp and 2.5 mAs. Process the image receptor.

4. Repeat steps 1 and 2. Label the first half "exposure #5" and expose using 96 kVp and 1 mAs. Label the second half "exposure #6" and expose using 106 kVp and 1 mAs. Process the image receptor.

5. Place a CR cassette on top of the radiographic table and center the hand phantom to the center of the cassette. Center and collimate the central ray to the hand and expose using 45 kVp, 8 mAs. Process the image using a hand algorithm and label the image "exposure #7."

6. Repeat step 5 using 55 kVp, 8 mAs for image 8; 73 kVp, 2 mAs for image 9; 83 kVp, 2 mAs for image 10; 96 kVp, 1 mAs for image 11; and 106 kVp, 1 mAs for image 12.

RESULTS

1. Review the screen/film and digital images with respect to radiographic IR exposure and image contrast.

LABORATORY 27-3 (Continued)

ANALYSIS

1. Is the background exposure similar on all three images?

2. For both the screen/film and digital images, which image demonstrates the lowest contrast? What is the reason for this?

3. For both the screen/film and digital images, which image demonstrates the highest contrast? What is the reason for this?

4. For both the screen/film and digital images, which image demonstrates the greatest difference between the contrast of the two exposures? Explain.

5. For both the screen/film and digital images, which image demonstrates the least difference between the contrast of the two exposures? Explain.

6. Summarize the effect that kVp has on exposure latitude, using the laboratory results to support your statements.

7. Explain the practical clinical application that is supported by the results of this laboratory activity.

LABORATORY 27-4 THE EFFECT OF GRIDS ON IMAGE CONTRAST

PURPOSE

Demonstrate the effectiveness of radiographic grids in the improvement of image contrast.

FOR FURTHER REVIEW

Refer to Chapter 27 in the accompanying textbook for further review of this topic.

MATERIALS

1. Energized radiographic unit

2. Image processor

3. Low- and high-ratio radiographic grids

4. Abdomen phantom

5. 14″ × 17″ image receptors

6. Step wedge (penetrometer)

7. Densitometer

SUGGESTED EXPOSURE FACTORS

200 mA, 0.03 sec, 75 kVp, 40″ SID, non-grid

PROCEDURES

1. Center the abdomen phantom to the image receptor (IR) on the tabletop. Place the step wedge beside the phantom on the IR. Direct the central ray perpendicular and collimate to the edges of the IR.

2. Using the suggested exposure factors, expose the image receptors, process, and label it "#1."

3. For film/screen image receptors, use a densitometer to measure the image receptors exposure of steps 4, 5, and 6 on the penetrometer and record the readings. The image receptor exposure of step 5 should be 1.2 ± 0.2. If not, adjust the mAs and re-expose.

4. Repeat the procedure using a low-ratio grid. Expose the image receptor using the appropriate grid conversion factor, process, and label it "#2."

5. Repeat the procedure using a high-ratio grid. Expose the image receptor using the appropriate grid conversion factor, process, and label it "#3."

6. Calculate the image contrast of each image by subtracting the image receptor exposure of step 6 from the OD of step 4.

7. For CR/digital image receptors, repeat steps 1 and 2. Expose the abdomen and process the image using the correct algorithm for an abdomen image.

LABORATORY 27-4 (Continued)

8. Use only the window width control to make the image completely light. Record this number. Carefully observe the effect on the demonstration of various structures as the window width is slowly increased to complete darkness. Record this number. Bring the window width back to the original number. Watch the monitor closely while the window width is very slowly increased. Record the number when the first visible change is observed.

RESULTS

1. Review the three images in terms of their exposure and contrast.

	Step Wedge Image Receptor Exposure			Contrast
	Step 4	Step 5	Step 6	Step 4 through Step 6
Image #1	_____	_____	_____	_____
Image #2	_____	_____	_____	_____
Image #3	_____	_____	_____	_____

ANALYSIS

1. Compare the image receptor exposure and image contrast of images 1, 2, and 3. Which image(s) more closely approximate(s) a quality image? Why?

2. Where are the differences in image contrast of the three images significant? Explain.

3. Based on your data, what conclusions can you draw about the effect of grids and grid ratio on image contrast?

4. What factors or influences have contributed to the decrease or increase of image quality in each of the images?

5. When using a digital imaging system, what effectively establishes the dynamic range of the image?

6. What visible image quality factor is changing as the window width is varied? Why is a radiographic grid important?

Name _____ Course _____ Date _____

 LABORATORY 28-1 THE EFFECT OF DISTANCE ON SPATIAL RESOLUTION

PURPOSE

Demonstrate the effects of object-to-image-receptor distance and source-to-image-receptor distance on spatial resolution.

FOR FURTHER REVIEW

Refer to Chapter 28 in the accompanying textbook for further review of this topic.

MATERIALS

1. Energized radiographic unit

2. 8″ × 10″ cassettes and image receptor

3. Dry bone parts

4. Radiolucent sponges, 2″ and 8″

5. Lead masks

6. Resolution test pattern

7. Image processor

SUGGESTED EXPOSURE FACTORS

1.0 mAs, 50 kVp, 40″ SID, non-grid

PROCEDURES

1. Mask a cassette in half and place the test pattern and a dry bone on a 2″ radiolucent sponge on the unmasked portion of the image receptor. Center the bone and test pattern to the unmasked half, label it "exposure #1," collimate to the edges of the unmasked area, and expose it using 50 kVp, 1 mAs, and 40″ SID.

2. Readjust the mask to the other half of the image receptor, center the bone and test pattern on top of an 8″ sponge on the unmasked portion of the cassette, label it "exposure #2," collimate to the unmasked area, expose it using the same technical factors, and process the image receptor.

3. Place a cassette on the floor, mask it in half and place the test pattern and dry bone on an 8″ radiolucent sponge on the unmasked portion of the cassette. Center the bone and test pattern to the unmasked half, label it "exposure #3," collimate it to the edges of the unmasked area, and expose it using 50 kVp and 60″ SID with the mAs adjusted according to the density maintenance formula (as derived from the inverse square law) to maintain the same density as the first image.

LABORATORY 28-1 (Continued)

RESULTS

1. Review all four images. Compare the spatial resolution of both the bone and the test pattern images. Carefully determine the image of the smallest group where the line pairs can be distinctly defined (separated) and record the lines/mm of the group below.

<u>Smallest Group Resolved (lines/mm)</u>

40″ SID/2″ OID   _____

40″ SID/8″ OID   _____

60″ SID/8″ OID   _____

ANALYSIS

1. Is there an obvious loss of recorded detail between the first two exposures of the bone? Which image demonstrates the best spatial resolution?

2. On exposures 1 and 2, is the spatial resolution loss as great in the test pattern as with the bone? Explain the reasons for the difference, if any. Indicate the greatest number of lines/mm demonstrated on each exposure.

3. Describe the spatial resolution of exposures 2 and 3. What is the greatest number of lines/mm that you can clearly see? What causes this difference? Explain.

4. Describe the effect of SID as it relates to image definition. Of what practical value is this knowledge to the radiographer?

5. Describe the advantage of high spatial resolution in digital imaging. What frequency signal does it represent?

Name _____ Course _____ Date _____

 LABORATORY 28-2 THE EFFECT OF FOCAL SPOT SIZE
ON SPATIAL RESOLUTION

PURPOSE

Demonstrate the effect of focal spot size on spatial resolution.

FOR FURTHER REVIEW

Refer to Chapter 28 in the accompanying textbook for further review of this topic.

MATERIALS

1. Energized radiographic unit

2. Image processor

3. CR processor

4. 8″ × 10″ image receptors

5. Dry bones

6. Resolution test pattern

7. Radiolucent sponge

SUGGESTED EXPOSURE FACTORS

100 mA, 0.01 sec, 50 kVp, 40″ SID, non-grid

PROCEDURES

1. Ascertain that the exposure factors to be used can be obtained with both a small and large focal spot. If not, locate a radiographic unit capable of satisfying this requirement.

2. Mask the IR in half, center a dry bone and the test pattern on a 2″ thick radiolucent sponge to the unmasked side, label it "exposure #1," and then collimate and expose it using the small focal spot.

3. Repeat step 2 on the other half of the image receptor, label it "exposure #2," expose it using the large focal spot, and process the image.

RESULTS

1. Review both images. Compare the spatial resolution of both the bone and the test pattern images. Carefully determine the image of the smallest group where the line pairs can be distinctly defined and record the lp/mm as follows.

Smallest Group Resolved (lp/mm)

Small Focal Spot   _____

Large Focal Spot   _____

LABORATORY 28-2 (Continued)

ANALYSIS

1. Is there an obvious loss of spatial resolution between the two images of the bone? Which image demonstrates the best resolution?

2. Is there an obvious loss of spatial resolution between the two resolution test patterns? Indicate the greatest number of lp/mm that you can see clearly defined in each of the images.

3. Is this loss as appreciable as that demonstrated in the images of the bones? Explain the reasons for your conclusion.

Name _____ Course _____ Date _____

 LABORATORY 28-3 THE EFFECT OF MOTION ON SPATIAL RESOLUTION

PURPOSE

Demonstrate the effect of object motion on spatial resolution.

FOR FURTHER REVIEW

Refer to Chapter 28 in the accompanying textbook for further review of this topic.

MATERIALS

1. Energized radiographic unit

2. CR image receptor

3. Hand phantom

4. String

SUGGESTED EXPOSURE FACTORS

See procedure

PROCEDURES

1. Mask an indirect digital cassette in half, center the hand phantom to the unmasked area, direct a perpendicular CR to the center of the hand, collimate to the unmasked section, and expose using 25 mA, 1.0 sec, 50 kVp, 500 SID, non-grid.

2. Remask to the other half and repeat step 1 with the hand in motion. Motion can be achieved by tying to the phantom a piece of string of sufficient length to reach the control booth and gently pulling the phantom during the exposure. (It is best to practice several times before making the exposure.)

RESULTS

1. Review both images. Consider the spatial resolution of each image.

ANALYSIS

1. Is there a difference in the spatial resolution of the two images? If a difference is noted, describe it.

2. Why does motion reduce spatial resolution?

LABORATORY 28-3 (Continued)

3. List the two types of patient motion associated with imaging. Give two methods that could be used to control each type.

LABORATORY 29-1 THE EFFECT OF DISTANCE ON SIZE DISTORTION

PURPOSE

Demonstrate the effect of OID and SID on size distortion.

FOR FURTHER REVIEW

Refer to Chapter 29 in the accompanying textbook for further review of this topic.

MATERIALS

1. Energized radiographic unit

2. Image processor

3. 10″ × 12″ image receptor

4. Small dry bone (vertebra preferred)

5. Metric ruler

SUGGESTED EXPOSURE FACTORS

100 mA, 0.01 sec, 50 kVp, 40″ SID, non-grid

PROCEDURES

OID Procedure

1. Mask an image receptor in quarters, center a dry bone on a 2″ thick radiolucent sponge to the unmasked area, label it "exposure #1," collimate, and expose.

2. Repeat step 1 on an unmasked area, using another sponge to increase the OID to 4″, label it "exposure #2," and expose.

3. Repeat step 1 on an unmasked area, using another sponge to increase the OID to 8″, label it "exposure #3," and expose.

4. Repeat step 1 on an unmasked area, using another sponge to increase the OID to 12″, label it "exposure #4," expose, and process.

SID Procedure

1. Mask an image receptor in quarters, center a dry bone on a 2″ thick radiolucent sponge to the unmasked area, change the SID to 20″, use the exposure maintenance formula (as derived from the inverse square law) to adjust the exposure factors, label it "exposure #5," collimate, and expose.

2. Repeat step 1 on an unmasked area using 30″ SID, use the exposure maintenance formula to adjust the exposure factors, label it "exposure #6," and expose.

LABORATORY 29-1 (Continued)

3. Repeat step 1 on an unmasked area using 40″ SID, use the exposure maintenance formula to adjust the exposure factors, label it "exposure #7," and expose.

4. Repeat step 1 on an unmasked area using 60″ SID (this distance is best obtained by placing the cassette on the floor), use the exposure maintenance formula to adjust the exposure factors, label it "exposure #8," expose, and process.

RESULTS

1. Accurately record the length of the dry bone and the images from the various exposures.

2. Calculate and record the magnification factor and percentage of magnification for each image.

OID DATA FORM

DRY BONE (OBJECT) LENGTH (OL) = _____ mm   SID = _____

OID	Bone Image Length (IL) (mm)	Magnification Factor (m) $\dfrac{SID}{SID - OID}$	% Magnification (% M) $\dfrac{IL - OL}{OL} \times 100$
2″			
4″			
8″			
12″			

SID DATA FORM

DRY BONE (OBJECT) LENGTH (OL) = _____ mm   OID = _____

SID	mAs	Bone Image Length (IL) (mm)	Magnification Factor (m) $\dfrac{SID}{SID - OID}$	% Magnification (% M) $\dfrac{IL - OL}{OL} \times 100$
20″				
30″				
40″				
60″				

LABORATORY 29-1 (Continued)

ANALYSIS

1. What happens to the recorded size of the image as the OID increases?

2. At what point does the loss of spatial resolution become unacceptable? Explain.

3. What happens to the recorded size of the image as the SID increases?

4. At what point does the loss of spatial resolution become unacceptable? Explain.

5. Describe the role of SID in producing size distortion and indicate how you would use this information to your advantage to produce an image with minimal size distortion.

6. Compare the results of the two procedures. Which factor produces the greatest influence on size distortion? Support your answer.

LABORATORY 29-1 (Continued)

7. Do the magnification factor and percentages compare favorably? Explain.

8. What effect does size distortion have on spatial resolution?

Name _____ Course _____ Date _____

LABORATORY 29-2 THE EFFECT OF ALIGNMENT AND ANGULATION ON SHAPE DISTORTION

PURPOSE

Demonstrate the effects of part/image receptor alignment, central ray/part/image receptor alignment, and central ray direction on shape distortion.

FOR FURTHER REVIEW

Refer to Chapter 29 in the accompanying textbook for further review of this topic.

MATERIALS

1. Energized radiographic unit

2. Image processor

3. 10″ × 12″ cassette with image receptor

4. Dry bone

5. Metric ruler

SUGGESTED EXPOSURE FACTORS

100 mA, 0.01 sec, 50 kVp, 40″ SID, non-grid

PROCEDURES

Part/Image Receptor Alignment

1. Position a 10″ × 12″ cassette lengthwise on the tabletop so the ID blocker is down, mask the cassette in thirds lengthwise, tape the dry bone on a 4″ sponge so that the long axis of the bone is parallel to the tube axis, center the bone to an unmasked area, direct the central ray to the center of the bone with a 40″ SID, label it "exposure #1," and expose.

2. Repeat step 1 on an unexposed area, center the bone to the area, direct the central ray to the center of the bone with a 40″ SID, raise the right (cathode) end of the sponge so the bone forms a 30° angle with the image receptor plane, label it "exposure #2," and expose.

3. Repeat step 1 on an unexposed area, center the bone to the area, direct the central ray to the center of the bone with a 40″ SID, raise the left (anode) end of the sponge so the bone forms a 30° angle with the image receptor plane, label it "exposure #3," expose, and process the receptor.

CR/Part/Image Receptor Alignment

1. Position a 10″ × 12″ image receptor (IR) lengthwise on the tabletop so the ID blocker is down, mask the IR in thirds lengthwise, tape the dry bone on a 4″ sponge so that the long axis of the bone is parallel to the tube axis, center the bone to an unmasked area, direct the central ray to the center of the bone with a 40″ SID, label it "exposure #4," and expose.

2. Repeat step 1 on an unmasked area, center the bone to the area, direct the central ray to the left (toward the anode) along the longitudinal axis of the bone until it is 6″ off-center, open the collimator to include the entire bone, label it "exposure #5," and expose.

3. Repeat step 1 on an unmasked area, center the bone to the area, direct the central ray to the right (toward the cathode) along the longitudinal axis of the bone until it is 6″ off-center, open the collimator to include the entire bone, label it "exposure #6," expose, and process the images.

Central Ray Direction

1. Position a 10″ × 12″ cassette lengthwise on the tabletop so the ID blocker is down, mask the cassette in thirds lengthwise, tape the dry bone on a 4″ sponge so that the long axis of the bone is parallel to the tube axis, center the bone to an unmasked area, direct the central ray to the center of the bone with a 40″ SID, label it "exposure #7," and expose.

2. Repeat step 1 on an unmasked area, center the bone to the area, direct the central ray to the left (toward the anode) along the longitudinal axis of the bone until it is 6″ off-center, angle back 25° to the original centering point, reduce the SID to 40″, label it "exposure #8," and expose.

3. Repeat step 2 on an unmasked area, direct the central ray to the right (toward the cathode) along the longitudinal axis of the bone until it is 6″ off-center, angle back 25° to the original centering point, reduce the SID to 40″, label it "exposure #9," expose, and process the receptor.

RESULTS

1. Accurately measure the length of the dry bone and the images of the bone on the image receptor and record them in mm.

Part/IR Alignment	Image 1	Image 2	Image 3
	_____	_____	_____
Central Ray/Part/IR Alignment	Image 4	Image 5	Image 6
	_____	_____	_____
Central Ray Direction	Image 7	Image 8	Image 9
	_____	_____	_____

ANALYSIS

Part/IR Alignment

Dry Bone Length _____ mm   Bone Image Length (mm)

1. Compare the differences in anatomical appearance between the recorded images in which portions are elongated/foreshortened. Compare image 1 to image 2, 1 to 3, and 2 to 3.

2. Can shape distortion caused by improper part/image receptor relationship also contribute to size distortion? Explain.

LABORATORY 29-2 (Continued)

3. To minimize shape distortion, indicate the most ideal relationship between the structures of interest and the film plane.

Central Ray/Part/Image Receptor Alignment

4. Compare the differences in anatomical appearance between the recorded images in which portions are elongated/foreshortened. Compare image 4 to image 5, 4 to 6, and 5 to 6.

5. Can shape distortion caused by improper central ray/part/IR alignment also contribute to size distortion? Explain.

6. Describe the significance of off-centering of the central ray to the visualization of joint spaces or nondisplaced fractures.

Central Ray Direction

7. Compare the differences in anatomical appearance between the recorded images in which portions are elongated/ foreshortened. Compare image 7 to image 8, 7 to 9, and 8 to 9.

8. Can shape distortion caused by improper central ray direction through the part also contribute to size distortion? Explain.

LABORATORY 29-2 (Continued)

9. Would it be more appropriate to direct the central ray perpendicular to the image receptor or to the structure of interest? Explain your answer and provide some practical examples that support your position.

10. Compare the shape distortion produced in the three different scenarios. Of the three causes of shape distortion identified, which produces the most obvious misrepresentation of the structure? Support your answer with examples.

11. Name three examinations/projections in which shape distortion is used to best advantage and describe how this is accomplished.

LABORATORY 30-1 IMAGE CRITIQUE: ASSESSING IMAGE RECEPTOR EXPOSURE, CONTRAST, SPATIAL RESOLUTION, AND DISTORTION

PURPOSE

Critique images effectively.

FOR FURTHER REVIEW

Refer to Chapter 30 in the accompanying textbook for further review of this topic.

MATERIALS

1. A repeated image

PROCEDURES

1. Use the procedures described in Chapter 30 of the textbook to critique the repeated images, using the following form.

ANALYSIS

IMAGE CRITIQUE FORM

I. CLASSIFY THE IMAGE AS:
☐ **WITHIN ACCEPTANCE LIMITS**

    ☐ Optimal diagnostic information (critique is complete)

<u>(all checkmarks below this line require completion of section II and III)</u>

    ☐ Suboptimal diagnostic information

☐ **OUTSIDE ACCEPTANCE LIMITS**

II. DETERMINE THE CAUSE OF THE PROBLEM AS:
☐   **A:**   **Technical Factors**

    ☐ Photographic problem with visibility of spatial resolution

      ☐ IR Exposure

        ☐ mAs_____

        ☐ Influencing factor (specify) _____

      ☐ Contrast

        ☐ Influencing factor (specify) _____

    ☐ Geometric problem with resolution

      ☐ Spatial resolution

        ☐ Geometry (specify) _____

        ☐ Image Receptor _____

        ☐ Motion _____

      ☐ Distortion

        ☐ Size (Magnification) (specify)_____

        ☐ Shape (Part/Image Receptor /Tube Alignment) (specify) _____

☐   **B:**   **Procedural Factors**

    ☐ Patient Positioning

      ☐ Tube Alignment _____

      ☐ Part Alignment _____

      ☐ Image Receptor Alignment _____

    ☐ Patient Preparation (specify) _____

☐   **C:**   **Equipment Malfunction**

    ☐ Processing Equipment (specify) _____

    ☐ Radiographic/Fluoroscopic Equipment (specify) _____

III. RECOMMENDED CORRECTIVE ACTION For each cause specified above:

_____

_____

_____

LABORATORY 31-1 ESTIMATING FOCAL SPOT SIZE

PURPOSE

Evaluate focal spot size using a star x-ray test pattern.

FOR FURTHER REVIEW

Refer to Chapter 31 in the accompanying textbook for further review of this topic.

MATERIALS

1. Energized radiographic unit

2. Image processor

3. 1.5- or 2-degree star x-ray test pattern

4. 10″ × 12″ image receptor

5. Small metric ruler

SUGGEST ED EXPOSURE FACTORS

5 mAs, 70 kVp, 24″ SID, non-grid

PROCEDURES

1. Locate the tube identification plate attached to the x-ray tube housing of the unit being tested. Record the nominal (manufacturer's specification) focal spot sizes that are indicated on the plate for the x-ray tube. They often appear as simply single decimal numbers (for example, 0.6 to 2.0 to indicate 0.6-mm and 2.0-mm focal spots).

2. Activate the collimator localizer light of the x-ray tube being evaluated, place the star test pattern in contact with the faceplate of the collimator so it is centered to the center, and rotate the star so one set of lead lines is parallel with the long axis of the tube and the other set is perpendicular. Tape the test pattern to the collimator faceplate in this position.

3. Center the image receptor lengthwise on the radiographic table, mask it in half crosswise, adjust the central ray perpendicular to the center of the unmasked area, label the anode and cathode sides of the image receptor, use a 24″ SID, collimate to the unmasked portion of the image receptor, select the large focal spot, and expose.

4. Readjust the mask, repeat step 2 using the small focal spot, expose, and process the image. An OD of 1.2 to 1.5 should be obtained if possible.

5. Determine the magnification (M) factor by dividing the diameter of the radiographic image of the star test pattern by the true diameter of the star test pattern.

6. Determine the point at which failure of resolution occurs. By viewing the image starting at the outer margin of the star pattern, move inward to the first area of blurring and mark this point. Mark the point where failure of resolution occurs on all four sides. Measure the distance in millimeters between the two marks along the anode cathode axis (D1) to determine the width of the focal spot. Measure the distance in millimeters between the two marks perpendicular to the anode cathode axis (D2) to determine the length of the focal spot.

7. Calculate the equivalent focal spot size (F_{mm}) according to the following formula:

$$F_{mm} = [N \div 57.3] \times [D \div (M - 1)]$$

where:

N = the angle of the star pattern used for the evaluation, that is, 1.5 or 2

D = distance between failure of resolution marks in mm

M = magnification factor

F_{mm} = equivalent focal spot size in mm

RESULTS

	Small Focal Spot	Large Focal Spot
Nominal Size	_____	_____
Equivalent Size	_____	_____

ANALYSIS

1. What are the measured equivalent sizes of the large and small focal spots?

2. How do these figures compare to the nominal (manufacturer specified) focal spot size for the tube evaluated?

3. Describe three other methods that can be used to evaluate focal spot size.

4. Describe the differences between effective, equivalent, and actual focal spot size.

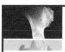 **LABORATORY 31-2** EVALUATING COLLIMATOR, CENTRAL RAY, AND BUCKY TRAY ALIGNMENT

PURPOSE

Evaluate the alignment of the light field and central ray to the x-ray beam and Bucky tray as well as the accuracy of the automatic collimation system.

FOR FURTHER REVIEW

Refer to Chapter 31 in the accompanying textbook for further review of this topic.

MATERIALS

1. Energized radiographic unit equipped with PBL
2. Image processor
3. Various size CR image receptors
4. One sheet of cardboard for each CR cassette size
5. Four paper clips
6. Collimator alignment template or nine pennies
7. X-ray beam perpendicularity test tool

SUGGESTED EXPOSURE FACTORS

25 mA, 0.05 sec, 50 kVp, 40″ SID, non-grid

PROCEDURES

Light Field X-Ray Beam Alignment and Perpendicularity

1. Center the alignment template on the IR and place it on the tabletop.
2. Center the light field to the cross centering mark on the template using 40″ SID.
3. Switch the PBL to manual mode and adjust the collimator light field to the field marks on the template.
4. If the light field is centered to the template, and one or more of the edges of the light field are not on the corresponding field marks, place straightened paper clips on the edges of the light field to mark the location.
5. Place the perpendicularity test tool on the template, making sure it is exactly centered to the template and to the center of the light field.
6. Place ID markers on the tabletop in the quadrant of the light field that represents the right shoulder of a supine patient (for orientation purposes in the event misalignment is noted) and expose the receptor.
7. Open the collimator to cover the entire receptor, expose a second time using half the mAs (this will be a double exposure), and process the image.
8. Evaluate the image for alignment of the x-ray beam to the light field.

Acceptance Limits

1. Federal guidelines for certified equipment allow ± 2 percent of the SID for alignment of the x-ray beam to the light field. The edges of the radiation field should be within ± 1 cm of the template markers indicating the location of the light field edges.

2. The image of the BBs in the perpendicularity test tool should appear within 5 mm of one another.

Nine-Penny Test for Beam Alignment

1. Center a $10'' \times 12''$ image receptor on the x-ray tabletop with its long dimension parallel to the long dimension of the table.

2. Center the light field to the center of the IR at a $40''$ SID.

3. Manually collimate the x-ray beam to a $6'' \times 8''$ field size.

4. Position two pennies in the center of each margin of the light field so that one entire penny is inside the light field and one is outside the light field. Place the ninth penny in the quadrant of the light field that represents the right shoulder of a supine patient as an orientation marker.

5. Place lead markers well inside the light field on the IR to identify the room number and date and expose the image receptor at about 50 kVp and 1.25 mAs.

6. Open the collimator and adjust the light field size to the IR and expose again using 50 kVp and 0.5 mAs (this will be a double exposure), and process the image.

7. Evaluate the accuracy of the x-ray field.

Acceptance Limits

Federal guidelines for certified equipment allow ± 2 percent of the SID for alignment of the x-ray to the light field. For a 100-cm ($40''$) SID, ± 2 cm (one penny) is acceptable. The alignment of x-ray to light field should be well within this guideline. Alignment to ± 1 cm (± 0.5 penny) can reasonably be achieved.

Field Size versus Image Receptor Size for Automatic Collimation (PBL) Systems

1. Set the x-ray tube at the usual source-to-image-receptor distance used for Bucky radiographs.

2. Set the PBL selector to the automatic mode.

3. Insert each size of image receptors commonly used in the Bucky tray lengthwise and then transversely. Visually check that the changes in the light field size occur with the changes in IR size and that the size of the light field is appropriate by comparing the light field size to the receptor size using scrap cardboard sheets.

Acceptance Limits

Federal guidelines for certified equipment allow ± 3 percent of the SID for PBL misalignment; however, a ± 1 cm is reasonably achievable.

LABORATORY 31-2 (Continued)

X-Ray Field and Bucky Alignment

1. Set the x-ray tube to the transverse center position.

2. Place straightened paper clips on the x-ray tabletop along the crosshairs of the collimator light field.

3. Insert a $10'' \times 12''$ image receptor lengthwise in the Bucky tray. Collimate the beam to an $8'' \times 10''$ size with the long dimension parallel to the x-ray tabletop.

4. Place ID markers on the tabletop in the quadrant of the light field that represents the right shoulder of a supine patient (for orientation purposes in the event misalignment is noted) and expose using about 50 kVp and 5 mAs.

5. Measure the distance from the center of the image as indicated by the crossed paper clips to the edges of the exposed portion of the image and to the edges of the receptor.

<u>Acceptance Limits</u>

The exposed portion of the image should be centered to the film within ± 1 cm in both length and width. The center indicated by the images of the crossed paper clips should actually be centered to the exposed portion of the image to within ± 1 cm.

RESULTS

1. Evaluate all of the test images against the acceptance criteria.

ANALYSIS

1. Was the radiation light field alignment within acceptable limits? Explain. Discuss the clinical implications of a misaligned radiation beam and light field.

2. Were the radiation beam centering and perpendicularity within acceptable limits? Explain. Discuss the clinical implications of misalignment of the center of the beam and a beam that is not perpendicular.

3. Was the PBL test within acceptable limits? If not, explain the unacceptable elements. Discuss the clinical implications of an improperly operating PBL device.

4. Was the Bucky tray beam center alignment within acceptable limits? Explain. Discuss the clinical implications of an improperly aligned Bucky tray.

5. List at least four causes of centering and radiation-to-light-field misalignment.

LABORATORY 31-3 EVALUATING DISTANCE, CENTERING, AND ANGULATOR ACCURACY

PURPOSE

Evaluate the accuracy of an SID indicator, centering detent, and angulation indicator.

FOR FURTHER REVIEW

Refer to Chapter 31 in the accompanying textbook for further review of this topic.

MATERIALS

1. Energized radiographic unit

2. Image processor

3. 8″ × 10″ CR with image receptor

4. Quarter or other coin

5. Ring stand

6. Paper sheet protector for a piece of 8 × 11 paper

7. Small ruler

8. Skull angulator or protractor

9. Small bubble level

SUGGESTED EXPOSURE FACTORS

100 mA, 0.0083 sec, 60 kVp, 40″ SID, 8:1 Bucky grid

PROCEDURES

SID Indicator Accuracy

1. Set up the ring stand on the tabletop 20″ above the Bucky tray and center it on the table. Cut a 4″ × 4″ section from a paper sheet protector and place it on the ring support. Center a quarter on the film, use the tube's SID indicator to position the tube 40″ above the Bucky tray, center the central tray to the quarter, and collimate appropriately. Place an 8″ × 10″ CR image receptor in the Bucky tray and center it to the central ray, expose, and process.

2. Use a metric ruler to determine the diameter of the quarter (object size). Measure the diameter of the image of the quarter on the test image (image size). Calculate the SID using the following equation:

$$SID = \frac{\text{Image size} \times \text{OID}}{\text{Image size} - \text{object size}}$$

Tube Centering Detent Accuracy

1. Place the x-ray tube at the center detent position and visually inspect the tube housing from the end and front of the table to make sure it is not angled (a bubble level can be used for more accuracy). Turn on the light localizer and note the position of the crosshairs on the tabletop. The longitudinal crosshair should be aligned to the midline of the table.

LABORATORY 31-3 (Continued)

Angulation Indicator Accuracy

1. Position the tube head so that the angulation indicator reads 0 degrees. Place the bubble level on top of the tube housing and determine if the bubble indicates a level tube position. Angle the tube in both directions and watch the indicator to see if it is accurate. A protractor or skull angulator can be used to verify the correct angle.

RESULTS

SID Indicator Accuracy

Indicated SID _____

Calculated SID _____

Angulation Indicator Accuracy

Angulation indicator reading
with tube head leveled _____

Tube Centering Detent Accuracy

Distance between crosshair
and table center line _____

ANALYSIS

1. What is the calculated SID?

2. The SID indicator should be within ±2 percent of the calculated SID to be considered accurate. What is the percentage difference between the indicated SID and the calculated SID? Does the SID indicator pass the accuracy test?

3. Did the light localizer crosshair align with the midline of the table with the tube in the detent position? If not, by how much was it off?

4. Assume that the table did not have a center line. Describe a way that could be used to determine the accuracy of the detent mechanism.

5. Did the angulation indicator read 0 degrees with the tube head in a level position? If not, by how much was it off?

6. Describe at least one adverse effect that could result from each of the three parameters if they tested as being inaccurate.

LABORATORY 31-4 EVALUATING KILOVOLTAGE ACCURACY

PURPOSE

Evaluate the accuracy of kVp production.

FOR FURTHER REVIEW

Refer to Chapter 31 in the accompanying textbook for further review of this topic.

MATERIALS

1. Energized radiographic unit

2. Image processor

3. Digital kVp meter

SUGGESTED EXPOSURE FACTORS

See procedure

PROCEDURES

Digital kVp Meter

1. The kVp settings evaluated should represent common kVp and mAs settings. Evaluate 60, 70, 80, 90, and 100 kVp at two different mA stations. If the generator is used for fluoroscopy, evaluate 120 instead of 60 kVp.

2. Set the meter for radiographic testing and for three-phase or single-phase depending on the type of generator. Most meters should be warmed up by an exposure of about 100 mAs and 100 kVp.

3. Position the meter on the table so the LCD readout is visible from the control booth, the detector is centered to the x-ray beam at 40″ source-to-detector distance, and collimate to approximately 6″ × 6″.

4. Set the desired kVp, use 100 ms or longer for three-phase generators and 200 ms or longer for single-phase generators (shorter exposure times [down to 50 ms] can be used without significant loss of accuracy), and expose.

5. Record the results. If no indication of sufficient intensity for a measurement occurs, decrease the source-to-detector distance or increase the mA. Do not change the kVp or time.

6. Repeat steps 3 through 5 for the remaining test exposures.

LABORATORY 31-4 (Continued)

RESULTS

Digital kVp Meter

1. Record the kVp meter readings below.

Tested kVp	mA	Measured kVp
_____	_____	_____
_____	_____	_____
_____	_____	_____
_____	_____	_____
_____	_____	_____

2. The kVp on a properly calibrated generator should be maintained within ± 2 kVp. A variation of ± 5 kVp or more should be corrected by a service engineer.

ANALYSIS

1. Were all the kVp settings tested within acceptable limits? If not, which ones were not and by how much?

2. Why is kVp considered such an important technical factor? Why must it be closely monitored?

3. What is the reason for aligning the long axis of the test cassette with the long axis of the x-ray tube?

4. How does accurate kVp impact EI values?

5. What are two possible causes of kVp variations?

LABORATORY 31-5 EVALUATING TIMER ACCURACY

PURPOSE

Evaluate the accuracy of an exposure timer.

FOR FURTHER REVIEW

Refer to Chapter 31 in the accompanying textbook for further review of this topic.

MATERIALS

1. Energized radiographic unit

2. Image processor

3. Digital exposure timer

4. 8″ × 10″ cassette with image receptor

5. Timer protractor template or ordinary protractor

SUGGESTED EXPOSURE FACTORS

2.5 mAs, 70 kVp, 40″ SID, non-grid

Digital X-Ray Exposure Timer (for All Types of Generators)

1. Turn the timer on. Select the appropriate measurement mode (Pulse—single phase, Time in sec, or Time in msec). Use the Time in sec mode for measuring times greater than 1/2 sec and the Time in msec for times less than 1/2 sec. Pulse mode will indicate the number of pulses delivered from a single-phase generator.

2. Position the meter level on the table so the LCD readout is visible from the control booth. The detector (indicated on the surface of the meter) is centered to the x-ray beam at a 40″ source-to-detector distance. Collimate to the area of the detector.

3. Set the kVp at 80 and mA at 200. Select an exposure time to be tested and make an exposure.

4. Record the results. If the meter displays obviously high or low values, notify your instructor.

5. Repeat steps 3 through 5 for three different exposure time settings for the remaining test exposures.

Acceptance Criteria

For three-phase generators, exposure time error should be limited to ± 5 %.

LABORATORY 31–5 (Continued)

RESULTS

Digital Exposure Timer

Time Station Tested	Measured Exposure Time
_____	_____
_____	_____
_____	_____
_____	_____

ANALYSIS

1. Were all the time stations evaluated within acceptable limits? If not, which ones were not and by how much?

2. What aspects of image quality are directly affected by exposure time?

Name _____ Course _____ Date _____

 LABORATORY 31-6 **EVALUATING EXPOSURE REPRODUCIBILITY, mA LINEARITY, AND mR/mAs**

PURPOSE

Evaluate the reproducibility and linearity of a generator for commonly used exposure settings.

FOR FURTHER REVIEW

Refer to Chapter 31 in the accompanying textbook for further review of this topic.

MATERIALS

1. Energized radiographic unit

2. Digital dosimeter

SUGGESTED EXPOSURE FACTORS

Choose an mAs that will produce dosimeter readings in the range of 200 to 500 mR at 80 kVp.

PROCEDURES

1. Turn on the digital dosimeter, select the dose mode, and follow the manufacturer's instructions for the unit's operation.

2. Place the dosimeter detector (ionization chamber) on the radiographic table and using a 40″ source-to-detector distance, center and collimate the beam to the detector.

3. On the generator control panel, select 80 kVp, 100 mA, and an exposure time that will result in a dosimeter reading between 200 and 500 mR. Readjust the exposure time if necessary until the reading is within this range and record the values.

4. Randomly change the technical factor settings and then go back to the desired setting. Make three exposures and record the readings on the data form as X_1, X_2, and X_3, respectively.

5. Repeat steps 3 and 4, but use the next larger mA station (i.e., 200 mA).

6. Repeat steps 3 and 4, but use the next larger mA station (i.e., 300 mA).

7. Repeat steps 3 and 4, but use the next larger mA station (i.e., 400 mA).

8. In order to properly analyze the results of this test, certain simple calculations must be made and the results compared to the acceptance criteria:

   a. Calculate the average of the three exposure measurements made at each kVp, mA, and time combination and record on the data form.

$$\text{Average } X = (X_1 + X_2 + X_3)/3$$

   b. Calculate the average exposure (Avg.) per indicated mAs for each mA and time station tested as:

$$\text{Avg. mR/mAs} = \text{Avg. } X/(mA \times s)$$

where: Average X is the average value of the recorded exposures at each mA and time station combination, and mA and s are the values of the stations selected. Record the calculated Avg. mR/mAs values on the data form.

c. For reproducibility, calculate and record on the data form the ratios X_1/Avg. X, X_2/Avg. X, and X_3/Avg. X for each kVp, mA, and time combination.

Acceptance Criteria

For any specific combination of selected technique factors, the exposures shall provide reproducible exposure to 0.05 or less. Thus, at a given kVp, mA, and time combination, the individual exposure measurements shall fall within 65 percent of the averages. This is indicated by X_n/Avg. X ratios between 0.95 and 1.05.

d. For linearity, use the calculated mR/mAs values to determine the linearity across all the mA stations selected at 80 kVp.

$$\text{Linearity} = [(\text{Avg. mR/mAs})_{max} - (\text{Avg. mR/mAs})_{min}]/[(\text{Avg. mR/mAs})_{max} + (\text{Avg. mR/mAs})_{min}]$$

where: $(\text{Avg. mR/mAs})_{max}$ and $(\text{Avg. mR/mAs})_{min}$ are the maximum and minimum values of the calculated mR/mAs as recorded on the data form.

Acceptance Criteria

Essentially, linearity means that the ratio of exposure to total charge in mR/mAs is constant over the entire range of mAs values. The average mR/mAs obtained at any tube current settings (mA) shall not differ by more than 0.10. Linearity should be maintained to ± 10 percent over the entire working range of the generator regardless of the number of mA stations at a fixed kVp.

9. Generator output is determined by taking the average of the four mR/mAs values. Average output produced by diagnostic x-ray equipment with a total filtration of 2.5 mm Al measured at 80 kVp with a 40″ source-to-detector distance should be 5.0 mR/mAs for single phase and 8.0 mR/mAs for three phase.

Acceptance Criteria

The tested generator should agree with the average values to within ± 30 percent, assuming other tests indicate proper performance, that is, kVp, SID accuracy, HVL, and so forth.

RESULTS

1. Document the results of the test and calculations in the appropriate sections of the data form.

DATA FORM

mA							
Time							
mAs							
X_1							
X_2							
X_3							
Avg. X							
X_1/Avg. X							
X_2/Avg. X							
X_3/Avg. X							
Avg. mR/mAs							

LABORATORY 31-6 (Continued)

ANALYSIS

1. Did the test results meet the acceptance criteria for reproducibility of the mA, linearity across mA stations, and output? If not, indicate which tests failed and support your conclusions.

2. Briefly discuss the importance of the reproducibility and linearity tests.

3. What might be a cause for reproducibility being unacceptable? Linearity?

4. Describe the benefits that can be derived from knowing the exposure output of the generators in an x-ray department. Why is exposure output expressed in mR/mAs?

Name _____ Course _____ Date _____

 LABORATORY 31-7 REJECTED-IMAGE STUDIES

PURPOSE

Analyze rejected images in a radiology department.

FOR FURTHER REVIEW

Refer to Chapter 31 in the accompanying textbook for further review of this topic.

MATERIALS

1. Images rejected during a survey period (A 4-week survey period is recommended)

2. Rejected image analysis worksheet

PROCEDURES

1. Set a start date and length for the survey period. At the end of the survey period, collect all rejected images (digital) and determine the total number of images used during this period.

2. Estimate the total number of images produced during the period of the study by multiplying the number of examinations by the average number of images produced per examination in each room.

3. Analyze the rejected images to determine the reason that they were probably rejected, using the categories listed on the rejected analysis worksheet.

RESULTS

1. Using the rejected analysis worksheet, record the number of images in each category against the exam type they represent according to the exam categories listed on the next page.

ANALYSIS

1. Calculate the rejected rate (%) based on the data collected for the survey period.

2. Calculate the rejected rate (%) of images by reason category.

3. List suggestions for corrective measures (actions) to minimize the repeat rates in the problem areas identified.

LABORATORY 31-7 (Continued)

REJECTED ANALYSIS WORKSHEET—PERCENTAGE BY ROOM

	1	2	3	4
REASON				
Overexposure				
Underexposure				
Positioning				
Centering				
Motion				
Other				
TOTAL				

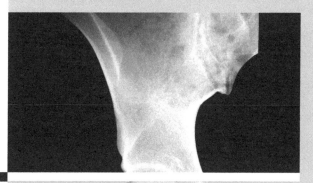

UNIT VI **Special Imaging Systems and Modalities**

LABORATORY 32-1 THE EFFECT OF ALIGNMENT AND DISTANCE ON MOBILE RADIOGRAPHIC IMAGE QUALITY

PURPOSE

Demonstrate the effect of central ray alignment and distance on image quality during mobile procedures.

FOR FURTHER REVIEW

Refer to Chapter 32 in the accompanying textbook for further review of this topic.

MATERIALS

1. Energized radiographic unit

2. Image processor

3. 10″ × 12″ Image receptor (IR)

4. Coconut (milk-filled) (when buying coconut, shake to hear milk)

SUGGESTED EXPOSURE FACTORS

100 mA, 0.05 sec, 5 mAs, 50 kVp, 40″ SID

PROCEDURES

Alignment Problems

1. Place the coconut in the center of the image receptor, direct the central ray to the center of the IR, collimate to the IR, set the tube to a 40″ SID, label the image "#1," expose, and process the image.

2. Place the IR in a vertical position, label the image "#2," and use a horizontal beam to repeat step 1 (use sponges as necessary to place the coconut in the center of the IR).

3. Place the IR at a 45° angle to the plane of the floor, label the image "#3," and use a horizontal beam to repeat step 1.

4. Place the IR at a 45° angle to the plane of the floor, label the image "#4," direct the central ray perpendicular to the IR, and repeat step 1.

Estimating Distance

1. Conceal the distance indicator on the radiographic unit, estimate a 36″ SID, then reveal the distance indicator and record the actual SID.

2. Repeat step 1 estimating 40″, 56″, and 72″ SIDs.

Distance/IR Exposure Problems

1. Place the coconut in the center of the IR, direct the central ray to the center of the IR, collimate to the IR, set the tube to a 36″ SID, label the image "#5," expose, and process.

2. Repeat step 1, using a 38″ SID for image 6, a 40″ SID for image 7, and a 42″ SID for image 8.

RESULTS

Estimating Distance

1. Record the actual distance for the following estimated distances:

   36″ SID   _____

   40″ SID   _____

   56″ SID   _____

   72″ SID   _____

ANALYSIS

Alignment Problems

1. Review images 1 through 4. Which of the images demonstrate a sharp air-fluid level within the coconut?

2. What is the proper procedure to demonstrate air-fluid levels in a patient?

3. What effects do image receptor and tube placement have on the demonstration of air-fluid levels?

Estimating Distance

4. How close were the actual distances to the estimated distances?

5. What effect will estimating distance for a mobile procedure have on image quality?

Distance/IR Exposure Problems

6. Review images 5 through 8. What effects do small changes in distance have on radiographic exposure?

7. How much of a distance change is necessary to notice the effect of the change on the image?

LABORATORY 33-1 FLUOROSCOPIC AUTOMATIC BRIGHTNESS CONTROLS

PURPOSE

Explain the effects of a fluoroscopic automatic brightness control on the image during fluoroscopy.

FOR FURTHER REVIEW

Refer to Chapter 33 in the accompanying textbook for further review of this topic.

MATERIALS

1. Stationary or mobile fluoroscopic unit

2. Lead apron

3. Large radiographic phantom (e.g., chest, abdomen, or pelvis)

EXPOSURE FACTORS

Suggested Factors

Medium mA (by setting brightness control) at 70 to 120 kVp

PROCEDURES

1. Only one individual should be within the fluoroscopic room during this experiment. Others shall be behind the protective barrier, near the control panel if using a stationary unit, and they shall observe and document the exposure conditions.

2. Wearing a lead apron, the individual within the fluoroscopic room should place the phantom at the center of the fluoroscopic unit and move the carriage into the operating position.

3. Use the foot pedal to activate the fluoroscope. Move the carriage until the phantom is centered to the image.

4. Move the carriage slowly from the center of the phantom to one side, observing the image closely during the motion.

5. Return the carriage slowly to the center of the phantom and then move it gradually up or down until the phantom disappears from the image.

6. Resume fluoroscopy again while observing the monitor. Open and close the collimators.

LABORATORY 33-1 (Continued)

ANALYSIS

1. Describe how the image changes as the fluoroscope moves from a thick portion of the phantom to a thin region.

2. Identify the mechanism that causes the changes described in question 1 and explain how it works.

3. What changes occurred in the image in terms of brightness, noise/fog, and contrast when the collimators were closed?

WORKSHEET 34-1 TOMOGRAPHY AND DIGITAL TOMOSYNSTHESIS

PURPOSE

Explain the tomographic principle and how 3-D mammography uses tomosynthesis to enhance mammographic imaging.

FOR FURTHER REVIEW

Refer to Chapter 34 in the accompanying textbook for further review of this topic.

ACTIVITIES

Answer the following questions:

1. Explain the tomographic principle.

2. Define *exposure amplitude* and describe its relationship to the tomographic section thickness.

3. Define *fulcrum* and describe its relationship to the focal plane.

4. How many exposures are required to establish an adequate image base for reprocessing in digital tomosynthesis?

5. In addition to breast imaging, tomosynthesis may also be useful in _____ and _____ radiography.

Name _____ Course _____ Date _____

WORKSHEET 35-1 MAMMOGRAPHY EQUIPMENT

PURPOSE
Explain differences between diagnostic radiography equipment and that specialized for mammography.

FOR FURTHER REVIEW
Refer to Chapter 35 in the accompanying textbook for further review of this topic.

ACTIVITIES
Answer the following questions:

1. What are the primary reasons for considering high-frequency generators for mammography?

2. What is the kVp range utilized in mammography?

3. Mammographic contrast must be sufficient to demonstrate microcalcifications that are extremely small. What is the size range that must be visualized adequately?

4. What is the major disadvantage of using kVp in the 20-s range?

5. What is the typical mammography mA range?

6. What materials are used for the target of mammography x-ray tube anodes?

7. What is the minimum HVL required by the U.S. government for 30 kVp?

8. What is the range of mammography grid ratios and frequencies?

9. Describe the process of digital tomosynthesis used in mammography.

Name _____ Course _____ Date _____

PURPOSE

Understand the imaging and equipment used for bone densitometry procedures.

FOR FURTHER REVIEW

Refer to Chapter 36 in the accompanying textbook for further review of this topic.

ACTIVITIES

Answer the following questions:

   1. What are the two basic bone types in the human body?

   2. How does the World Health Organization define how far a patient's BMD is deviated from the mean of a sex-matched young adult population reaching its peak bone mass?

   3. Which body part should be scanned when the patient presents with a diagnosis of hyperparathyroidism?

   4. Define the term *precision* and describe how it affects the equipment used for bone densitometry.

5. Using the image below, match the following anatomical structures with the letters on the image.

_____   Lesser trochanter

_____   Neck of femur

_____   Ischium

_____   Trochanteric region

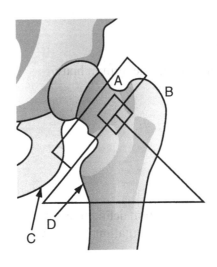

Name _____ Course _____ Date _____

PURPOSE

Describe the imaging equipment used for specialized vascular and interventional radiologic procedures.

FOR FURTHER REVIEW

Refer to Chapter 37 in the accompanying textbook for further review of this topic.

ACTIVITIES

Answer the following questions:

1. What are the three digital image acquisition modes used in vascular imaging? Explain the common uses for each mode.

2. What post-processing functions can be used to compensate for patient motion?

3. Why is a C-arm assembly commonly used in vascular imaging instead of a traditional fluoroscopic image intensification unit?

4. What are the five factors that affect injector flow rate?

WORKSHEET 38-1 COMPUTED TOMOGRAPHY

PURPOSE

Explain the basic features of computed tomographic units and the basic acquisition and display methods used in CT.

FOR FURTHER REVIEW

Refer to Chapter 38 in the accompanying textbook for further review of this topic.

ACTIVITIES

Answer the following questions:

   1. What technology allows for the use of helical scanning methods in CT?

   2. Explain the term *multisection CT* (MSCT) and explain the significance of this development in CT scanning.

   3. List the major components of a computed tomographic unit.

   4. List the three parameters that determine detector dose efficiency.

   5. Briefly explain how Hounsfield units are calculated and specify the HUs associated with air, water, and bone.

6. What is a convolution filter?

7. Describe the relationship between the voxel, pixel, and matrix size in terms of image resolution.

8. What are the most common artifacts and their causes encountered in CT imaging?

9. List two parameters used to determine patient dose in CT imaging.

WORKSHEET 39-1 MAGNETIC RESONANCE IMAGING

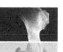

PURPOSE

Explain the basic function of magnetic resonance imaging (MRI) units, including the basic acquisition and display methods used in MRI.

FOR FURTHER REVIEW

Refer to Chapter 39 in the accompanying textbook for further review of this topic.

ACTIVITIES

Answer the following questions:

1. What is the Larmor frequency and why is it critical to MRI?

2. Identify the primary parameters controlling the MRI process. Compare and contrast these parameters.

3. What purpose do gradient coils serve in acquiring an MR image? How many gradient coils are necessary to obtain an image, and why?

4. What role do radiofrequency pulse sequences play in obtaining various MR images?

5. Highlight the key safety factors associated with MRI.

LABORATORY 39-2 EVALUATING MAGNETIC RESONANCE IMAGES

PURPOSE

Evaluate basic parameters of an MR image.

FOR FURTHER REVIEW

Refer to Chapter 39 in the accompanying textbook for further review of this topic.

MATERIALS

1. Images from a complete abdominal MRI examination with essentially normal anatomy imaged in transverse, sagittal, and coronal images
2. Images from a complete abdominal CT examination with essentially normal anatomy (MRI and CT images may be from different patients)

ANALYSIS

1. Locate the following structures on transverse, sagittal, and coronal sections:
   a. Vertebral body
   b. Liver
   c. Kidney
   d. Aorta
   e. Vena cava

2. Name an area that appears dark as a result of a signal void.

3. Describe the differences in the image of a vertebral body on the MR image as compared to the CT image.

4. Describe the differences in the image of muscles on the MR image as compared to the CT image.

WORKSHEET 40-1 NUCLEAR MEDICINE EQUIPMENT

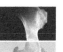

PURPOSE

Explain the basic function of nuclear medicine (NM) equipment, including the basic acquisition and display methods used in NM.

FOR FURTHER REVIEW

Refer to Chapter 40 in the accompanying textbook for further review of this topic.

ACTIVITIES

Answer the following questions:

1. Describe a parallel collimator and how the transmission of photons occurs.

2. Identify the operational parameters controlling SPECT imaging. Compare and contrast these parameters.

3. Describe the major components of a gamma camera.

4. Compare PET and SPECT imaging and describe the advantages of each.

5. Explain the concept of hybrid imaging and give an example.

LABORATORY 40-2 EVALUATING NUCLEAR MEDICINE IMAGES

PURPOSE

Analyze NM images.

FOR FURTHER REVIEW

Refer to Chapter 40 in the accompanying textbook for further review of this topic.

MATERIALS

1. Normal NM bone scan

2. Abnormal NM bone scan

ANALYSIS

1. Locate the following structures on both images:

   a. Spine

   b. Liver

   c. Kidney

   d. Femur

   e. Pelvis

2. Name an area that appears dark as a result of increased isotope uptake.

3. Compare any differences in the images in the area of the lumbar spine.

4. Describe the differences in the images of the femurs.

WORKSHEET 41–1 RADIATION THERAPY

PURPOSE

Explain the basic function of radiation therapy, including the difference between image fusion and hybrid imaging.

FOR FURTHER REVIEW

Refer to Chapter 41 in the accompanying textbook for further review of this topic.

ACTIVITIES

Answer the following questions:

1. Describe the responsibilities of a dosimetrist.

2. Describe the difference between structural imaging methods and functional imaging methods.

3. Define gross tumor volume (GTV), clinical target volume (CTV), and planning target volume (PTV). How are these important in treatment planning?

4. What role does image-guided radiation therapy (IGRT) play in tumor location?

5. List the five components of a linear accelerator.

Name_____ Course _____ Date _____

PURPOSE

Analyze ultrasound images.

FOR FURTHER REVIEW

Refer to Chapter 42 in the accompanying textbook for further review of this topic.

ACTIVITIES

Answer the following questions:

IMAGE #1

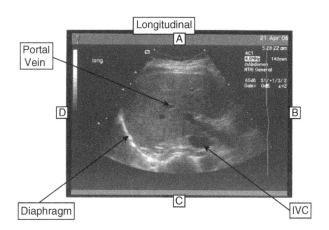

1. Label the orientation for A, B, C, and D.

    A _____

    B _____

    C _____

    D _____

2. The IVC is _____ to the diaphragm.

3. The portal vein is _____ to the IVC.

4. The diaphragm is _____ to the portal vein.

IMAGE #2

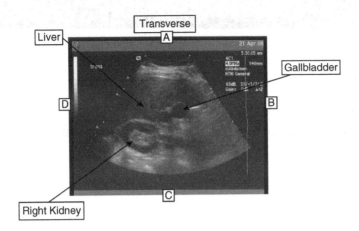

1. Label the orientation for A, B, C, and D.

   A _____

   B _____

   C _____

   D _____

2. The liver is _____ to the right kidney.

3. The gallbladder is to the _____ of the liver.

4. The right kidney is _____ and to the _____
   of the gallbladder.

Name _____ Course _____ Date _____

PURPOSE

Analyze Doppler images.

FOR FURTHER REVIEW

Refer to Chapter 42 in the accompanying textbook for further review of this topic.

ACTIVITIES

IMAGE #1

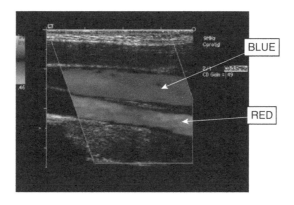

1. The color blue indicates what type of Doppler shift, positive or negative? Explain why.

2. The color red indicates what type of Doppler shift, positive or negative? Explain why.

3. The above image depicts a common carotid artery and a jugular vein. Which color represents the common carotid artery and which represents the jugular vein?

4. Is the common carotid artery showing flow going toward the transducer or away from the transducer? Explain why.

5. Is the jugular vein showing flow going toward the transducer or away from the transducer? Explain why.

6. Which vessel will have a reflected wave with higher frequency, the red or blue?

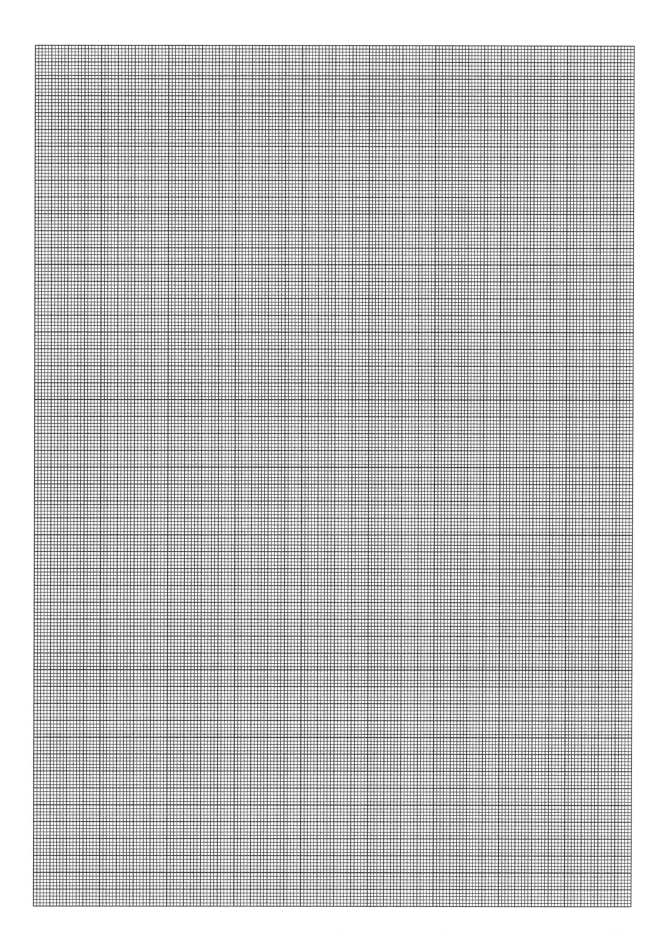

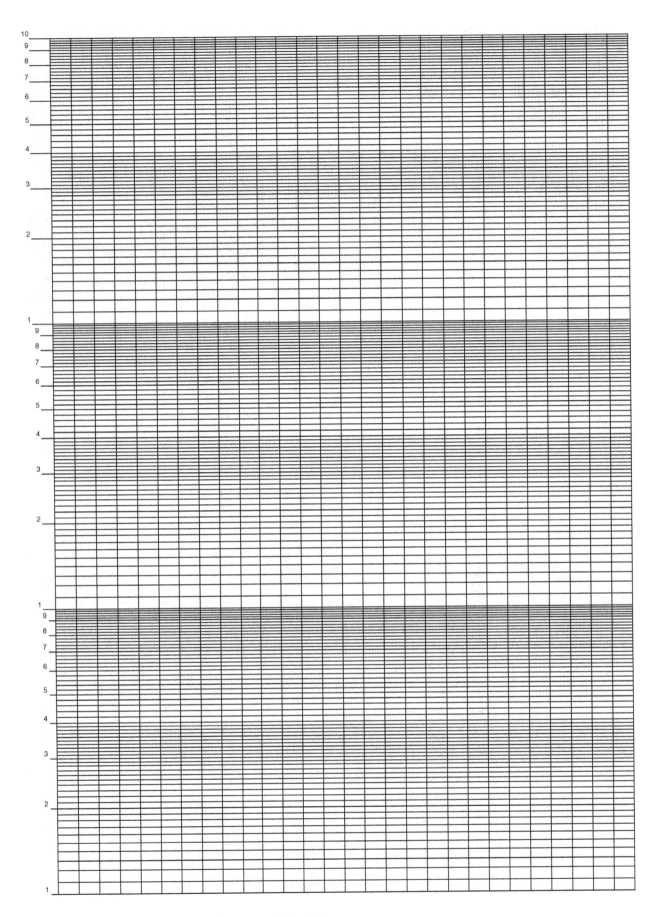

Notes

Notes

Notes

Notes

Notes

Notes